D0422742

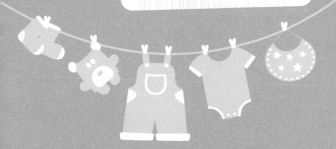

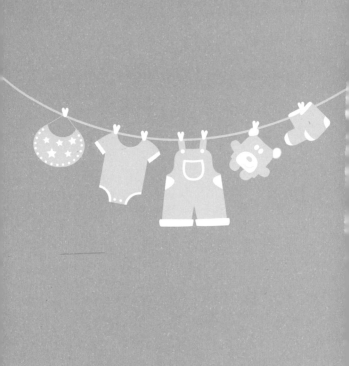

BABY
Names

BABY NAMES

Summersdale Publishers Ltd
46 West Street
Chichester
West Sussex
PO19 1RP
UK

www.summersdale.com

Printed and bound in China

ISBN: 978-1-84953-370-6

Substantial discounts on bulk quantities of Summersdale books are available to corporations, professional associations and other organisations. For details contact Nicky Douglas by telephone: +44-(0)1243-756902, fax: +44-(0)1243-786300 or email: nicky@summersdale.com.

BABY
Names

Choosing the perfect
name for your little star

Emily Harper

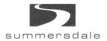

summersdale

Contents

Activists

Actors (Film)

Actors (Television)

Animators

Architects

Artists

Astronauts

Astronomers

Aviators

Ballet Dancers

Basketball Players

Bassists

Biologists

Boxers

Celebrity Offspring

Chefs

Chemists

Child Actors

Comedians

Composers

Computer Scientists

Cricketers

Diarists

Drummers

Ecologists

Engineers

Entrepreneurs

Explorers

Fashion Designers

Film Directors

Footballers

Gods (Greek)

Gods (Roman)

Golfers

Guitarists

Historians

Illustrators

Inventors

Journalists

Lawyers

Magicians

Mathematicians

Military Leaders

Monarchs (Ancient)

Monarchs (Modern)

Mountaineers

Olympians (Summer)

Olympians (Winter)

Paralympians

Philosophers

Photographers

Physicists

Pianists

Playwrights

Poets

Political Leaders

Psychologists

Racing Drivers

Radio Personalities

Rappers

Religious Leaders

Rugby Players

Shakespearean Characters

Singers (Jazz)

Singers (Opera)

Singers (Pop)

Singers (Rock)

Spies

Talk Show Hosts

Teachers

Tennis Players

Violinists

Writers

Writers (Children's)

Zoologists

Activists

Alva Belmont
1853–1933, American women's rights activist

Daisy Bates
1914–1999, American civil rights leader

Emmeline Pankhurst
1858–1928, English leader of the suffragette movement

Florence Kelley
1859–1932, American children's rights campaigner

Harriet Tubman
1820–1913, African-American Civil War spy and abolitionist

Joy Adamson
1910–1980, Austrian author of *Born Free*

Michelle Bachelet
Born 1951, Chilean human rights activist and president

Pearl Buck
1892–1973, American activist for civil and women's rights

Rosa Parks
1913–2005, African-American 'first lady of civil rights'

Sheila Rowbotham
Born 1943, English feminist theorist and writer

Activists

Asa Philip Randolph
1889–1979, founded first industrial union for African Americans

Bayard Rustin
1912–1987, American activist for civil rights, pacifism, non-violence and gay rights

Ciro Alegría
1909–1967, Peruvian human rights activist and author

Eugene Debs
1855–1926, American, organised first industrial union

Jackson Browne
Born 1948, German environmental and anti-war activist

Malcolm X
1925–1965, African-American human rights activist

Martin Luther King Jr
1929–1968, African-American leader of civil rights movement

Sidney Hillman
1887–1946, Lithuanian–American campaigner for employment rights

Stokely Carmichael
1941–1998, Trinidadian–American civil rights activist

William Du Bois
1868–1963, African-American civil rights campaigner

Actors (film)

Angelina Jolie
Born 1975, American actor and director

Audrey Hepburn
1929–1993, Oscar-winning British screen legend

Helen Mirren
Born 1945, Oscar-winning English actor

Ingrid Bergman
1915–1982, Oscar-winning Swedish–American screen legend

Judy Garland
1922–1969, American actor and singer

Marilyn Monroe
1926–1962, American Hollywood superstar

Naomi Watts
Born 1968, British–Australian actor

Octavia Spencer
Born 1970, Oscar-winning American actor

Sissy Spacek
Born 1949, Oscar-winning America actor and singer

Winona Ryder
Born 1971, American actor and producer

Actors (film)

Anthony Hopkins
Born 1937, Oscar-winning Welsh actor

Brad Pitt
Born 1963, American actor and producer

Christopher Lee
Born 1922, influential English actor

Donald Sutherland
Born 1935, Canadian actor

Gene Kelly
1912–1996, American actor, dancer and singer

Heath Ledger
1979–2008, Oscar-winning Australian actor and director

Hugh Grant
Born 1960, English actor and producer

Laurence Olivier
1907–1989, Oscar-winning decorated English screen legend

Leonardo DiCaprio
Born 1974, American actor and producer

Sean Connery
Born 1930, Oscar-winning Scottish actor

Actors (television)

Angela Lansbury
Born 1925, English *Murder, She Wrote* star

Courteney Cox
Born 1964, American star of *Friends*

Elizabeth Montgomery
1933–1995, American *Bewitched* actor

Evangeline Lilly
Born 1979, Canadian star of *Lost*

Letitia Dean
Born 1967, English *EastEnders* actor

Holly Valance
Born 1983, Australian singer and star of *Neighbours*

Jane Leeves
Born 1961, English star of *Frasier*

Rhea Perlman
Born 1948, American star of *Cheers*

Sofia Vergara
Born 1972, Columbian star of *Modern Family*

Zoë Wanamaker
Born 1949, American-born English TV and stage actor

Actors (television)

Ashton Kutcher
Born 1978, American star of *That '70s Show*

Christopher Lilley
Born 1974, Australian *Angry Boys* star

Dexter Fletcher
Born 1966, English star of *Band of Brothers*

Dominic West
Born 1969, English actor in *The Wire*

Henry Winkler
Born 1945, American, aka 'the Fonz' in *Happy Days*

Idris Elba
Born 1972, English, central character in *Luther*

Kelsey Grammar
Born 1955, American star of *Frasier*

Kiefer Sutherland
Born 1966, Canadian star of *24*

Sylvester McCoy
Born 1943, Scottish, seventh Doctor in *Doctor Who*

Ted Danson
Born 1947, American star of *Cheers*

Animators

Arlene Klasky
Born 1949, American co-founder of Klasky-Csupo

Elizabeth Case Zwicker
1930–2006, American, first female Disney animator

Faith Hubley
1924–2001, American Oscar-winning animator

Jennifer Yuh Nelson
Born 1972, South Korean–American animation director of *Kung Fu Panda*

Kazuko Nakamura
Born 1934, early female Japanese animator

Laverne Harding
1905–1984, American, Walter Lantz studio animator

Lillian Friedman
1912–1989, American, brought Popeye and Betty Boop to life

Lotte Reiniger
1899–1981, German, first female animator

Phyllis Barnhart
1922–2008, American Disney animator

Reiko Okuyama
1935–2007, pioneering Japanese animé artist

Animators

Hayao Miyazaki
Born 1941, Japanese co-founder of Studio Ghibli

Joseph Barbera
1911–2006, American co-founder of Hanna-Barbera

Matt Groening
Born 1954, American creator of *The Simpsons* and *Futurama*

Mike Judge
Born 1962, American creator of *Beavis and Butt-head*

Nick Park
Born 1958, English stop-motion animator, creator of *Wallace and Gromit*

Seth MacFarlane
Born 1973, American creator of *Family Guy*

Tex Avery
1908–1980, American creator of Bugs Bunny and Daffy Duck

Trey Parker
Born 1969, American co-creator of *South Park*

Walt Disney
1901–1966, legendary American animator and producer

William Hanna
1910–2001, American, other half of Hanna-Barbera

Architects

Anne Tyng
1920–2011, Chinese geometric architect

Denise Scott Brown
Born 1931, African-born American urban architect

Eileen Gray
1878–1976, Influential Irish architect

Julia Morgan
1872–1957, American designer of Hearst Castle

Kazuyo Sejima
Born 1956, award-winning Japanese architect

Marion Mahony Griffin
1871–1961, American, first ever licensed female architect

Maya Lin
Born 1959, American designer of Vietnam Veterans Memorial

Norma Merrick Sklarek
1928–2012, African-American designer of Terminal 1, Los Angeles International Airport

Susana Torre
Born 1944, Argentinian-born American architect and educator

Zaha Hadid
Born 1950, award-winning Iraqi–British architect

Architects

Alvar Aalto
1898–1976, Finnish architect and designer

Antoni Gaudí
1852–1926, Catalan modernist architect

Charles-Édouard Jeanneret
1887–1965, French pioneer of modern architecture, aka Le Corbusier

Frank Gehry
Born 1929, Canadian–American deconstructivist

Gordon Kaufmann
1888–1949, British-born American, designer of the Hoover Dam

Ieoh Ming Pei
Born 1917, Chinese–American abstract architect, designer of the Louvre Pyramid

Louis Sullivan
1856–1924, American 'father of modern architecture'

Norman Foster
Born 1935, English breakthrough architect, designer of 'The Gherkin'

Oscar Niemeyer
Born 1907, Brazilian designer of first modernist skyscraper

Santiago Calatrava
Born 1951, Spanish architect and sculptor

Artists

Artemisia Gentileschi
1593–1656, Italian Baroque painter

Bridget Riley
Born 1931, English optical artist

Eva Hesse
1936–1970, German–American sculptor

Frida Kahlo
1907–1954, Mexican surrealist artist

Joan Mitchell
1925–1992, American abstract-expressionist artist

Lavinia Fontana
1552–1614, Italian portrait artist

Louise Bourgeois
1911–2010, French–American contemporary artist

Marguerite Gérard
1761–1837, French painter and etcher

Marlene Dumas
1953–present, South African portrait artist

Natalia Goncharova
1881–1962, Russian avant-garde artist

Artists

Damien Hirst
Born 1965, Turner Prize-winning English artist

Edgar Degas
1834–1917, French impressionist artist

Giovanni Antonio Canal
1697–1768, Italian landscape painter, aka Canaletto

Henri Matisse
1869–1954, French fauvist artist

Leonardo da Vinci
1452–1519, Italian Renaissance artist and polymath

Lucian Freud
1922–2011, German-born British portrait artist

Michelangelo Merisi da Caravaggio
1571–1610, Italian Baroque painter

Pablo Picasso
1881–1973, Spanish cubist artist

Raffaello Sanzio da Urbino
1483–1520, Italian painter and architect, aka Raphael

Rembrandt Harmenszoon van Rijn
1606–1669, Dutch painter and etcher

Astronauts

Chiaki Mukai
Born 1952, first Japanese woman in space

Claudie Haigneré
Born 1957, first French woman in space

Eileen Collins
Born 1956, American, first female shuttle pilot

Helen Sharman
Born 1963, first Briton in space

Peggy Whitson
Born 1960, American, NASA's most experienced female astronaut

Roberta Bondar
Born 1945, first Canadian woman in space

Sally Ride
1951–2012, first American woman in space

Sunita Williams
Born 1965, American, longest female space flight

Svetlana Savitskaya
Born 1948, Russian, first woman to spacewalk

Valentina Tereshkova
Born 1937, Russian, first woman in space

Astronauts

Alexei Leonov
Born 1934, Russian, first human to spacewalk

Bruce McCandless II
Born 1937, conducted first untethered spacewalk

Buzz Aldrin
Born 1930, American, second person on the moon

Gherman Stepanovich Titov
1935–2000, Russian, the youngest person in space

James Lovell
Born 1928, American commander of Apollo 13

Neil Armstrong
1930–2012, American, first person on the moon

Story Musgrave
Born 1935, American astronaut and physician

Valery Polyakov
Born 1942, Russian, holds record for longest space flight

Wubbo Ockels
Born 1946, first Dutch person in space

Yuri Gagarin
1934–1968, Russian, first human in space

Astronomers

Agnes Mary Clerke
1842–1907, Irish astronomer and writer

Annie Jump Cannon
1863–1941, American developer of stellar classification

Caroline Herschel
1750–1848, German–British, discovered several comets

Cecilia Payne
1900–1979, British–American revelatory astronomer

Henrietta Swan Leavitt
1868–1921, posthumously influential American astronomer

Hypatia
*c.*351–415, Greek teacher of astronomy

Maria Mitchell
1818–1889, American discoverer of comets

Mary Somerville
1780–1872, Scottish astronomer and mathematician

Vera Rubin
Born 1928, respected American astronomer

Wendy Freedman
Born 1957, Canadian–American director of Carnegie Observatories

Astronomers

Arno Penzias
Born 1933, Nobel Prize-winning German–American astronomer

Charles Messier
1730–1817, French publisher of early astronomical catalogue

Claudius Ptolemy
c.90–168, Greco–Roman astronomer and geographer

Edwin Hubble
1889–1953, influential American cosmologist

Galileo Galilei
1564–1642, Italian astronomer and 'father of modern science'

Hipparchus
c.190–120 BC, Greek astronomer and geographer

Johannes Kepler
1571–1630, German, devised laws of planetary motion

Nicolaus Copernicus
1473–1543, revolutionary Polish Renaissance astronomer

Tycho Brahe
1546–1601, Danish astronomer and alchemist

William Herschel
1738–1822, German–British astronomer and composer

Aviators

Adrienne Bolland
1895–1975, French, first woman to fly over Andes

Amelia Earhart
1897–1937, American, first woman to fly solo across Atlantic

Amy Johnson
1903–1941, English record-breaking pilot

Bessica Raiche
1875–1932, American, first woman to fly a plane solo

Beverly Burns
Born 1949, American, first woman to captain a Boeing 747

Harriet Quimby
1875–1912, American, first woman to fly across English Channel

Melitta Schiller
1903–1945, decorated German Luftwaffe pilot

Pancho Barnes
1901–1975, American, first female stunt pilot

Polly Vacher
Born 1944, English long-distance aviator

Raymonde de Laroche
1882–1919, French, first woman to receive pilot's licence

Aviators

Anthony LeVier
1913–1998, American air racer and test pilot

Charles Lindbergh
1902–1974, American aviator and inventor

Erich Hartmann
1922–1993, German ace fighter pilot

Jacques-Étienne Montgolfier
1745–1799, French co-inventor of hot air balloon

James Doolittle
1896–1993, pioneering American aviator

Joseph Christopher McConnell Jr
1922–1954, top American flying ace

Manfred von Richthofen
1892–1918, German ace fighter pilot, aka 'The Red Baron'

Noel Wien
1899–1977, American founder of first Alaskan airline

Orville Wright
1871–1948, American co-inventor of first successful aeroplane

Wilbur Wright
1867–1912, American, other half of the Wright Brothers

Ballet Dancers

Adeline Genée
1878–1970, Danish–British world-famous ballet dancer

Anna Pavlova
1881–1931, Russian ballet legend

Cynthia Gregory
Born 1946, American ballet dancer and choreographer

Darcey Bussell
Born 1969, English, Principal Dancer with the Royal Ballet

Galina Ulanova
1910–1998, one of Russia's greatest ballerinas

Gelsey Kirkland
Born 1952, American star of the New York City Ballet

Lydia Kyasht
1885–1959, Russian prima ballerina

Margot Fonteyn
1919–1991, English ballet legend

Polina Semionova
Born 1984, Russian, one of the youngest ever prima ballerinas

Tamara Karsavina
1885–1978, Russian star of the Imperial Russian Ballet

Ballet Dancers

Ayman Safiah
Born 1991, Palestinian ballet dancer

Carlos Acosta
Born 1973, Cuban ballet star

Fernando Bujones
1955–2005, influential American dancer

Irek Mukhamedov
Born 1960, Russian Bolshoi Ballet dancer

Patrick Bissell
1957–1987, American ballet star

Pierre Vladimiroff
1893–1970, Russian dancer and teacher

Rudolf Nureyev
1938–1993, Russian ballet legend

Vadim Muntagirov
Born 1990, Russian, English National Ballet principal

Vaslav Nijinsky
1890–1950, Russian, early en pointe dancer

Yuri Soloviev
1940–1977, Russian dancer at the Kirov Ballet

Basketball Players

Azania Stewart
Born 1989, British international player

Carol Blazejowski
Born 1956, American medal winner

Cheryl Miller
Born 1964, American player, coach and commentator

Denise Curry
Born 1959, successful American player and coach

Hortência Marcari
Born 1959, influential Brazilian player

Lidia Alexeyeva
Born 1924, medal-winning Russian player and coach

Lynette Woodard
Born 1959, American, first female in Harlem Globetrotters

Sandra Kay Yow
1942–2009, successful American coach

Stef Collins
Born 1982, experienced British international player

Teresa Edwards
Born 1964, award-winning American player and coach

Basketball Players

Charles Barkley
Born 1963, American forward and sports analyst

Dražen Dalipagić
Born 1951, influential Yugoslavian player

Forrest Allen
1885–1974, successful American player and coach

Joel Freeland
Born 1987, English NBA player

Kareem Abdul-Jabbar
Born 1947, American all-time leading scorer

Kobe Bryant
Born 1978, American, Los Angeles Lakers shooting guard

Larry Bird
Born 1956, successful American player and coach

Meadowlark Lemon
Born 1932, American, 'Clown Prince' of the Harlem Globetrotters

Michael Jordan
Born 1963, iconic American shooting guard

Shaquille O'Neal
Born 1972, former American centre and rapper

Bassists

Aimee Mann
Born 1960, American singer-songwriter

D'arcy Wretzky
Born 1968, American, former Smashing Pumpkins bassist

Debbie Googe
Born 1962, English, My Bloody Valentine bassist

Gina Birch
Born 1955, English, member of The Raincoats

Jennifer Finch
Born 1966, American, bassist with L7

Juliana Hatfield
Born 1967, American singer-songwriter

Kim Gordon
Born 1953, American, Sonic Youth bassist

Melissa Auf der Maur
Born 1972, Canadian, Hole bassist

Shingai Shoniwa
Born 1981, English frontwoman of Noisettes

Suzi Quatro
Born 1950, American rock icon

Bassists

Cliff Burton
1962–1986, legendary Metallica four-stringer

Dusty Hill
Born 1949, American, ZZ Top bassist and co-vocalist

Geddy Lee
Born 1953, Canadian, Rush frontman

Harvey Bainbridge
Born 1949, English, Hawkwind bassist

Jaco Pastorius
1951–1987, American jazz musician

John Entwistle
1944–2002, English bassist with The Who

Lemmy
Born 1945, British Motörhead frontman

Paul McCartney
Born 1942, English singer-songwriter and musician, member of the 'Fab Four'

Phil Lynott
1949–1986, Irish frontman of Thin Lizzy

Rustee Allen
Born 1953, American member of Sly & the Family Stone

Biologists

Anne McLaren
1927–2007, English scientist, paved way for IVF

Barbara McClintock
1902–1992, American Nobel Prize-winning cytogeneticist

Christiane Nüsslein-Volhard
Born 1942, German Nobel Prize winner

Gerty Cori
1896–1957, Czech–American Nobel Prize winner

Jane Goodall
Born 1934, English primatologist and anthropologist

Maria Sibylla Merian
1647–1717, German naturalist and scientific illustrator

Mary Anning
1799–1847, pioneering English palaeontologist

Molly Stevens
Born 1974, English biomedical scientist and professor

Rachel Carson
1907–1964, American marine biologist

Sidnie Manton
1902–1979, English insect specialist

Biologists

Charles Darwin
1809–1882, English, proponent of the theory of evolution

Francis Crick
1916–2004, English co-discoverer of DNA molecular structure

George Simpson
1902–1984, American palaeontologist

Gregor Mendel
1822–1884, German founder of genetics

James Watson
Born 1928, American geneticist and co-discoverer of DNA molecular structure

Jean-Baptiste Lamarck
1744–1829, French evolutionary naturalist

Richard Dawkins
Born 1941, English author of *The Selfish Gene*

Ronald Fisher
1890–1962, English evolutionary biologist

Sewall Wright
1889–1988, American geneticist and evolutionary theorist

Theodosius Dobzhansky
1900–1975, Ukrainian geneticist and evolutionary biologist

Boxers

Bonnie Canino
Born 1962, American world featherweight champion

Daisy Lang
Born 1972, Bulgarian bantamweight world champion

Deirdre Gogarty
Born 1969, Irish featherweight world champion

Diana Dutra
Born 1964, Canadian junior world welterweight champion

Elena Reid
Born 1981, American world flyweight champion

Freeda Foreman
Born 1976, American middleweight, and daughter of George Foreman

Isra Girgrah
Born 1971, Yemeni world lightweight champion

Nicola Adams
Born 1982, English, Olympic gold medallist

Para Draine
Born 1972, American world flyweight and super flyweight champion

Rain Mako
Born 1976, glamorous New Zealand fighter

Boxers

Archie Moore
1916–1998, American light heavyweight world champion

Carlos Monzón
1942–1995, Argentinian middleweight world champion

Cassius Clay
Born 1942, American heavyweight and Olympic champion, aka Muhammad Ali

Evander Holyfield
Born 1962, American cruiserweight and heavyweight world champion

Frank Bruno
Born 1961, English, heavyweight world champion

George Foreman
Born 1949, American heavyweight champion and grill maker

Henry Cooper
1934–2011, decorated British heavyweight champion

Joe Frazier
1944–2011, American, Olympic gold medallist and world heavyweight champion

Lennox Lewis
Born 1965, British–Canadian heavyweight world and Olympic champion

Rocky Marciano
1923–1969, American, undefeated world heavyweight champion

Celebrity Offspring

Apple Martin
Born 2004, English, daughter of Gwyneth Paltrow and Chris Martin

Coco Cox Arquette
Born 2004, American, daughter of Courteney Cox and David Arquette

Destry Spielberg
Born 1996, American, daughter of Steven Spielberg

Lourdes Maria Ciccone Leon
Born 1996, American, daughter of Madonna

Memphis Eve Hewson
Born 1991, Irish, daughter of Bono

Moon Unit Zappa
Born 1967, American, daughter of Frank Zappa

Peaches Geldof
Born 1989, British, daughter of Bob Geldof and Paula Yates

Phoenix Chi Gulzar
Born 1999, English–Dutch daughter of former Spice Girl Mel Brown

Sonnet Whitaker
Born 1996, American, daughter of Forest Whitaker

Zuma Rossdale
Born 2008, British–American, daughter of Gwen Stefani and Gavin Rossdale

Celebrity Offspring

Banjo Taylor
Born 2003, Australian, son of Rachel Griffiths

Brooklyn Beckham
Born 1999, English, son of David and Victoria Beckham

Denim Braxton-Lewis
Born 2001, American, son of Toni Braxton

Geronimo James
Born 2004, English, son of Alex James

Kyd Duchovny
Born 2002, American, son of David Duchovny

Maddox Jolie
Born 2001, Cambodian–American, son of Angelina Jolie and Brad Pitt

Pirate Davis
Born 2005, American, son of Jonathan Davis (frontman of metal band Korn)

Sage Moonblood Stallone
1976–2012, American, son of Sylvester Stallone

Satchel Farrow
Born 1987, American, son of Woody Allen and Mia Farrow

Zowie Bowie
Born 1971, English, son of David Bowie

Chefs

Anjum Anand
Born 1971, English chef, champion of Indian cuisine

Delia Smith
Born 1941, English, doyenne of British cookery

Elena Arzak
Born 1969 award-winning Spanish chef

Fanny Cradock
1909–1994, theatrical English chef

Hélène Darroze
Born 1967, Michelin-starred French chef

Isabella Beeton
1836–1865, English Victorian cookery legend

Julia Child
1912–2004, France-loving American chef

Léa Linster
Born 1955, award-winning Luxembourgian chef

Lorraine Pascale
Born 1973, British model turned chef

Nigella Lawson
Born 1960, English chef, sex symbol and 'domestic goddess'

Chefs

Alain Ducasse
Born 1956, Michelin-starred Monégasque chef

Antonio Carluccio
Born 1937, Italian chef and restaurateur

Fergus Henderson
Born 1963, offal-loving English chef

Heston Blumenthal
Born 1966, experimental English chef

Joël Robuchon
Born 1945, French 'Chef of the Century'

José Andrés
Born 1969, America-based Spanish chef

Keith Floyd
1943–2009, eccentric English chef

Marco Pierre White
Born 1961, British celebrity chef

Raymond Blanc
Born 1949, French chef and renowned restaurateur

Valentine Warner
Born 1972, English chef and TV presenter

Chemists

Carolyn Bertozzi
Born 1966, American designer of artificial bones

Dorothy Hodgkin
1910–1994, English, developer of protein crystallography

Ellen Swallow Richards
1842–1911, American industrial and environmental chemist

Hazel Bishop
1906–1998, American, invented smear-proof lipstick

Irène Joliot-Curie
1897–1956, Nobel Prize-winning French chemist

Joan Berkowitz
Born 1931, American chemist and environmentalist

Louise Hammarström
1849–1917, Swedish mineral chemist

Marie Daly
1921–2003, African-American biochemist

Ruth Erica Benesch
1925–2000, American biochemist

Vera Popova
1867–1896, Russian ketone researcher

Chemists

Alfred Nobel
1833–1896, Swedish, invented dynamite and devised Nobel prizes

Amedeo Avogadro
1776–1856, Italian molecular theorist

Antoine Lavoisier
1743–1794, pioneering French chemist

Dmitri Mendeleyev
1834–1907, Russian, devised the Periodic Table

Friedrich Wöhler
1800–1882, German 'father of organic chemistry'

Henry Cavendish
1731–1810, English, theoretical chemist, discovered hydrogen

Irving Langmuir
1881–1957, American, high-temperature chemist

Jöns Jacob Berzelius
1779–1848, Swedish, developed chemical symbols

Josiah Willard Gibbs
1839–1903, American founder of chemical thermodynamics

William Perkin
1838–1907, English, discovered first aniline dye

Child Actors

Anna Paquin
Born 1982, Canadian-born New Zealand actor and Oscar winner

Deanna Durbin
Born 1921, Canadian child star

Drew Barrymore
Born 1975, American, sprang to fame in *ET*

Jodie Foster
Born 1962, American, made her name in *Taxi Driver*

Maureen McCormick
Born 1956, American known for role in *The Brady Bunch*

Natalie Wood
1938–1981, American Hollywood child star

Petula Clark
Born 1932, English child actor and singer

Ramona Marquez
Born 2001, British *Outnumbered* child actor

Raven-Symoné Pearman
Born 1985, American child star of *The Cosby Show*

Shirley Temple
Born 1928, legendary American child star

Child Actors

Brad Renfro
1982–2008, young American Hollywood actor

Christian Bale
Born 1974, British Hollywood child star

Corey Feldman
Born 1971, American, young star of the 1980s

Fred Savage
Born 1976, American, rose to fame in *The Wonder Years*

Gary Coleman
1968–2010, American child star of *Diff'rent Strokes*

Macaulay Culkin
Born 1980, famous American *Home Alone* star

Mickey Rooney
Born 1920, American whose career spans his lifetime

Neil Patrick Harris
Born 1973, American, star of *Doogie Howser, M.D.*

Roddy McDowall
1928–1998, English child actor

Sean Astin
Born 1971, American star of *The Goonies*

Comedians

Ellen DeGeneres
Born 1958, American comedian and TV host

Jenny Eclair
Born 1960, English comedian and novelist

Jo Brand
Born 1957, award-winning English comedian

Joan Rivers
Born 1933, brash American comedian

Nina Conti
Born 1974, English comedian and ventriloquist

Roseanne Barr
Born 1952, American sitcom actor and comedian

Ruby Wax
Born 1953, American alternative comedian and mental health campaigner

Sarah Silverman
Born 1970, American satirical comedian and musician

Shappi Khorsandi
Born 1973, Iranian-born British comedian

Victoria Wood
Born 1953, English actor and comic heroine

Comedians

Bill Hicks
1961–1994, respected American stand-up comedian

Dara Ó Briain
Born 1972, Irish comedian and TV host

Denis Leary
Born 1957, American actor and comedian

Dylan Moran
Born 1971, Irish actor and stand-up comedian

Eddie Izzard
Born 1962, bilingual English comedian and actor

Eric Morecambe
1926–1984, English, half of Morecambe and Wise

Frankie Boyle
Born 1972, pessimistic Scottish comedian

Rhod Gilbert
Born 1968, award-winning Welsh comedian

Richard Pryor
1940–2005, American actor and comedian

Steve Martin
Born 1945, multi-talented American performer

Composers

Amy Beach
1867–1944, first successful female American composer

Augusta Read Thomas
Born 1964, American composer and professor

Clara Schumann
1819–1896, German Romantic composer

Fanny Mendelssohn
1805–1847, German pianist and composer

Judith Weir
Born 1954, award-winning British composer

Kaija Saariaho
Born 1952, Finnish chamber and opera composer

Libby Larsen
Born 1950, Grammy-winning American composer

Ruth Crawford Seeger
1901–1953, American modernist composer

Sofia Gubaidulina
Born 1931, mould-breaking Russian composer

Chen **Yi**
Born 1953, Chinese composer and violinist

Composers

Edward Elgar
1857–1934, celebrated English composer

Frédéric Chopin
1810–1849, Polish composer and virtuoso pianist

George Frederick Handel
1685–1759, German–British Baroque composer

Giuseppe Verdi
1813–1901, Italian Romantic composer

Iannis Xenakis
1922–2001, Greek composer and music theorist

Johann Sebastian Bach
1685–1750, multi-talented German Baroque composer

Joseph Haydn
1732–1809, Austrian composer and father of the symphony

Karlheinz Stockhausen
1928–2007, experimental German composer

Ludwig van Beethoven
1770–1827, ground-breaking German composer

Wolfgang Amadeus Mozart
1756–1791, Austrian composer and child prodigy

Computer Scientists

Ada Lovelace
1815–1852, English, considered world's first computer programmer

Anita Borg
1949–2003, influential American computer scientist

Audrey Tang
Born 1981, Taiwanese free software programmer

Éva Tardos
Born 1957, Hungarian Fulkerson Prize winner

Grace Hopper
1906–1992, pioneering American computer scientist

Grete Hermann
1901–1984, German developer of computerised algebra

Hedy Lamarr
1913–2000, Austrian–American actor and wireless communications pioneer

Mary Lou Jepsen
Born 1965, American founder of Pixel Qi

Shafi Goldwasser
Born 1958, Israeli–American, co-invented zero-knowledge proofs

Sophie Wilson
Born 1957, English, designed Acorn Micro-Computer

Computer Scientists

Alan Turing
1912–1954, English 'father of computer science'

Bjarne Stroustrup
Born 1950, Danish creator of C++ programming language

Charles Babbage
1791–1871, English, developed concept of programmable computer

Edgar Codd
1923–2003, English, creator of Relational Database Model

Edsger Dijkstra
1930–2002, award-winning Dutch computer scientist

Edwin Catmull
Born 1945, American, president of Walt Disney and Pixar

John McCarthy
1927–2011, American, coined the term 'artificial intelligence'

Leonard Adleman
Born 1945, American co-inventor of the RSA cryptosystem

Tim Berners-Lee
Born 1955, English inventor of World Wide Web

Vinton Gray Cerf
Born 1943, American 'father of the Internet'

Cricketers

Belinda Clarke
Born 1970, groundbreaking Australian international

Betty Wilson
1921–2010, Australian, great all-round test player

Debbie Hockley
Born 1962, New Zealand captain

Janette Brittin
Born 1959, record-breaking England international

Johmari Logtenberg
Born 1989, South African test cricketer

Karen Rolton
Born 1974, Australian record holder for total runs scored

Mithali Raj
Born 1982, Indian international captain

Myrtle Maclagan
1911–1993, Indian-born English scorer of first test century in women's cricket

Rachel Heyhoe-Flint
Born 1939, captained England to win first Women's Cricket World Cup

Sana Mir
Born 1986, Pakistani international captain

Cricketers

Adam Gilchrist
Born 1971, Australian international wicket-keeper-batsman

Brian Lara
Born 1969, record-breaking West Indian international

Donald Bradman
1908–2001, Australian, considered the greatest batsman of all time

Garfield Sobers
Born 1936, West Indies, one of the greatest ever all-rounders

Imran Khan
Born 1952, Pakistan cricket captain and politician

Jacques Kallis
Born 1975, South African all-rounder

Sachin Tendulkar
Born 1973, superior Indian batsman

Shane Warne
Born 1969, Australian, one of the greatest ever bowlers

Viv Richards
Born 1952, West Indian, one of Wisden's five 'Cricketers of the Century'

Walter Hammond
1903–1965, England test captain

Diarists

Anaïs Nin
1903–1977, French–Cuban diarist and author

Anne Frank
1929–1945, German diarist and Holocaust victim

Aya Kito
1962–1988, teenage Japanese diarist

Celia Fiennes
1662–1741, English traveller and writer

Charlotte Forten Grimké
1837–1914, African-American anti-slavery activist

Hana Maria Pravda
1916–2008, Czech Holocaust survivor, actor and diarist

Hedvig Elisabeth Charlotte of Holstein-Gottorp
1759–1818, Swedish queen and famed diarist

Käthe Kollwitz
1867–1945, German artist and writer

Marjorie Fleming
1803–1811, Scottish child writer and poet

Violet Bonham Carter
1887–1969, English politician and diarist

Diarists

Alan Bennett
Born 1934, English playwright, author and actor

Alastair Campbell
Born 1957, English political aide and diarist

Allen Ginsberg
1926–1997, American beat poet and writer

Derek Jarman
1942–1994, English artist and author

Edmund C. Hinde
1830–1909, American gold miner and diarist

Francis Scott Fitzgerald
1896–1940, American novelist and diarist

Luca Landucci
1436–1516, Italian apothecary and diarist

Nicholas Blundell
1669–1737, English aristocrat and diarist

Rutherford Birchard Hayes
1822–1893, American president and diarist

Samuel Pepys
1633–1703, British politician famous for his diaries

Drummers

Carla Azar
Born 1987, American singer and drummer in Autolux

Evelyn Glennie
Born 1965, Scottish virtuoso percussionist

Honey Lantree
Born 1943, English, Honeycombs drummer

Janet Weiss
Born 1965, American drummer with Sleater-Kinney and Wild Flag

Karen Carpenter
1950–1983, American singer and drummer in The Carpenters

Maureen 'Moe' Tucker
Born 1944, American, Velvet Underground percussionist

Meg White
Born 1974, American, one half of The White Stripes

Paloma McLardy
Born 1955, Spanish drummer for The Slits and The Raincoats

Sandy West
1959–2006, American singer and drummer with The Runaways

Terri Lyne Carrington
Born 1965, award-winning American jazz drummer

Drummers

Buddy Rich
1917–1987, American virtuoso jazz drummer

Cozy Powell
1947–1998, prolific British rock drummer

Dave Grohl
Born 1969, American, Nirvana drummer and Foo Fighters frontman

Ginger Baker
Born 1939, English drummer for Cream and Blind Faith

John Bonham
1948–1980, English, legendary Led Zeppelin drummer

Keith Moon
1946–1978, English drumming hero with The Who

Nicko McBrain
Born 1952, English, Iron Maiden drummer

Ringo Starr
Born 1940, English, one quarter of the 'Fab Four'

Travis Barker
Born 1975, American, Blink-182 drummer

Zach Hill
Born 1979, unconventional American drummer

Ecologists

Celia Hunter
1919–2001, American environmental activist

Inés Mendoza
1908–1990, Puerto Rican First Lady and ecologist

Julia Butterfly Hill
Born 1974, American environmental campaigner

Lois Gibbs
Born 1951, American environmental activist

Pamela Matson
Born 1953, American ecologist and professor

Rachel Carson
1907–1964 American, revealed 'dark side' of science

Rosalie Edge
1877–1962, American conservationist

Ruth Patrick
Born 1907, American, developed new fieldwork techniques

Vandana Shiva
Born 1952, Indian environmental activist

Wangari Maathai
1940–2011, Kenyan social environmentalist

Ecologists

Alan Chadwick
1909–1980, English promoter of organic gardening

Aldo Leopold
1887–1948, American godfather of wilderness conservation

Archie Belaney
1888–1938, British–Canadian nature writer, aka 'Grey Owl'

Chico Mendes
1944–1988, Brazilian, rainforest campaigner

Eugene Odum
1913–2002, American, devised concept of ecosystems

Gifford Pinchot
1865–1946, American forester and conservationist

Gordon Orians
Born 1932, American ecologist and ornithologist

Jacques Cousteau
1910–1997, French oceanographer, conservationist and explorer

John Muir
1838–1914, Scottish-born American creator of modern ecology movement

Nicholas Hughes
1962–2009, British–American stream salmonid ecologist

Engineers

Edith Clarke
1883–1959, American electrical engineer and professor

Elsie Eaves
1898–1983, American civil engineer

Emily Roebling
1843–1903, American, chief engineer of Brooklyn Bridge construction

Hertha Ayrton
1854–1923, English engineer and inventor

Judith Resnik
1949–1986, American, NASA engineer and astronaut

Kayleigh Messer
Born 1986, English, Formula 1 motorsport engineer

Lillian Gilbreth
1878–1972, American industrial engineer

Nora Stanton Blatch Barney
1883–1971, British–American civil engineer and architect

Olive Dennis
1885–1957, revolutionary American railway engineer

Sarah Guppy
1770–1852, English, patented suspension bridge foundations

Engineers

Archimedes
c.287 BC–c.212 BC, Greek–Sicilian engineer, physicist and inventor

Edwin Armstrong
1890–1954, American inventor of the FM radio

George Stephenson
1781–1848, English 'Father of the Railways'

Gustave Eiffel
1832–1923, French engineer behind the Eiffel Tower

Isambard Kingdom Brunel
1806–1859, much-revered British civil engineer

James Watt
1736–1819, Scottish engineer, improved the steam engine

John Logie Baird
1888–1946, Scottish engineer, created first practical television

Nicolaus Otto
1832–1891, German inventor of internal-combustion engine

Seymour Cray
1925–1996, American electrical engineer and supercomputer architect

Willis Carrier
1876–1950, American inventor of modern air conditioning

Entrepreneurs

Anita Roddick
1942–2007, English founder of The Body Shop

Cher Wang
Born 1958, Taiwanese co-founder of the HTC Corporation

Doris Fisher
Born 1932, American co-founder of Gap

Estée Lauder
1908–2004, American co-founder of the eponymous cosmetics company

Florence Nightingale Graham
1884–1966, Canadian–American founder of Elizabeth Arden

Giuliana Benetton
Born 1937, Italian co-founder of Benetton

Jacqueline Gold
Born 1960, English chief executive of Ann Summers

Martha Lane Fox
Born 1973, English co-founder of Lastminute.com

Sheryl Sandberg
Born 1969, American, number two at Facebook

Yelena Baturina
Born 1963, Russian founder of the Inteco construction company

Entrepreneurs

Asa Candler
1851–1929, American founder of the Coca-Cola company

Berry Gordy Jr
Born 1929, American founder of Motown Records

Conrad Hilton Sr
1887–1979, American founder of Hilton Hotels

Elon Musk
Born 1971, South African-born American founder of PayPal

Henry Ford
1863–1947, American founder of the Ford Motor Company

Levi Strauss
1829–1902, German-born American creator of blue jeans

Mark Zuckerberg
Born 1984, American creator of Facebook

Narayana Murthy
Born 1946, Indian software engineer and co-founder of Infosys Technologies

Richard Branson
Born 1950, English creator of Virgin brand

Sergey Brin
Born 1973, Russian-born American co-founder of Google

Explorers

Annie Smith Peck
1850–1935, American mountaineer

Felicity Aston
Born 1977, English, first woman to ski alone across Antarctica

Freya Stark
1893–1993, English explorer and travel writer

Gertrude Bell
1868–1926, English explorer, archaeologist and spy

Gudridur Thorbjarnardóttir
Born c.980, Icelandic explorer of the west

Harriet Chalmers Adams
1875–1937, American explorer of South America, Asia and the South Pacific

Hester Stanhope
1776–1839, English explorer of the Holy Land

Kira Salak
Born 1971, American adventurer and journalist

Mary Kingsley
1862–1900, English explorer and ethnographer

Nellie Bly
1864–1922, record-breaking American explorer and journalist

Explorers

Christopher Columbus
1451–1506, Genoan New World explorer

Ernest Shackleton
1874–1922, Anglo–Irish polar explorer

Ferdinand Magellan
1480–1521, Portuguese explorer of Asia

Francisco Vásquez de Coronado
1510–1554, Spanish explorer of Mexico

Hernando De Soto
1496–1542, Spanish, first European to cross the Mississippi

James Cook
1728–1779, first Briton to travel to Australia

Marco Polo
1254–1324, Venetian explorer of Asia

Ranulph Fiennes
Born 1944, English, considered the greatest living explorer

Robert Falcon Scott
1868–1912, English, Antarctic explorer

Vasco da Gama
c.1460–1524, Portuguese explorer of India

Fashion Designers

Betsey Johnson
Born 1942, American whimsical fashion designer

Coco Chanel
1883–1971, French fashion legend

Donatella Versace
Born 1955, Italian vice president of the Versace empire

Elsa Schiaparelli
1890–1973, Italian surrealist-inspired designer

Jeanne Paquin
1869–1936, forward-thinking French designer

Phoebe Philo
Born 1973, French-born British designer

Stella McCartney
Born 1971, English designer and environmentalist

Tamara Mellon
Born 1967, English co-founder of Jimmy Choo

Vera Wang
Born 1949, American haute couture designer

Vivienne Westwood
Born 1941, English punk and new wave fashion designer

Fashion Designers

Alexander McQueen
1969–2010, English designer and couturier

Calvin Klein
Born 1942, American fashion icon

Christian Dior
1905–1957, French fashion legend

Domenico Dolce
Born 1958, Sicilian half of Dolce & Gabbana

Gianni Versace
1946–1997, Italian founder of the international fashion house

Giorgio Armani
Born 1934, Italian menswear designer

Jimmy Choo
Born 1952, Malaysian–Chinese shoe designer

Louis Vuitton
1821–1892, French businessman and designer

Valentino Garavani
Born 1932, Italian designer and founder of the world-famous Valentino brand

Yves Saint Laurent
1936–2008, French fashion legend

Film Directors

Debra Granik
Born 1963, American director of *Winter's Bone*

Jane Arden
1927–1982, Welsh director of *Anti-Clock*

Kathryn Bigelow
Born 1951, American director of *The Hurt Locker*

Lisa Cholodenko
Born 1964, American director of *The Kids Are All Right*

Lucile Hadzihalilovic
Born 1961, French director of *Innocence*

Lynne Ramsay
Born 1969, Scottish director of *We Need to Talk About Kevin*

Mimi Leder
Born 1952, American director of *Deep Impact*

Nancy Meyers
Born 1949, American director of *What Women Want*

Penelope Spheeris
Born 1945, American director of *Wayne's World*

Sofia Coppola
Born 1971, American director of *Lost in Translation*

Film Directors

Alfred Hitchcock
1899–1980, English director of *Psycho*

Francis Ford Coppola
Born 1939, American director of *The Godfather*

Ingmar Bergman
1918–2007, Swedish writer and director of *The Seventh Seal*

Orson Welles
1915–1985, American director and star of *Citizen Kane*

Quentin Tarantino
Born 1963, American director of *Pulp Fiction*

Ridley Scott
Born 1937, English director of *Blade Runner*

Stanley Kubrik
1928–1999, American director of *A Clockwork Orange*

Steven Spielberg
Born 1946, American director of *Jaws*

Werner Herzog
Born 1942, German director of *The Enigma of Kaspar Hauser*

Woody Allen
Born 1935, American director of *Annie Hall*

Footballers

Abby Wambach
Born 1980, American, Olympic gold medallist

Birgit Prinz
Born 1977, German World Cup winner

Cristiane Rozeira de Souza Silva
Born 1985, Brazilian forward

Hanna Ljungberg
Born 1979, Swedish forward

Homare Sawa
Born 1978, Japanese FIFA World Player of the Year

Kelly Smith
Born 1978, English forward

Marta Vieira da Silva
Born 1986, Brazilian forward

Mia Hamm
Born 1972, American FIFA World Player of the Year

Renate Lingor
Born 1975, German midfielder

Sun **Wen**
Born 1973, Chinese striker

Footballers

Bobby Moore
1941–1993, English World Cup winner

Clint Dempsey
Born 1983, American midfielder

Cristiano Ronaldo
Born 1985, Portuguese star

David Beckham
Born 1975, English football superstar

Diego Maradona
Born 1960, Argentinian legend

Eden Hazard
Born 1991, Belgian attacking midfielder

Fernando Torres
Born 1984, Spanish striker

George Best
1946–2005, Northern Irish, legendary Manchester United winger

Lionel Messi
Born 1987, Argentinian, Golden Shoe and Ballon d'Or winner

Rio Ferdinand
Born 1978, English centre-back

Goddesses (Greek)

Aphrodite
Goddess of love

Athena
Goddess of wisdom

Demeter
Goddess of fertility and harvest

Gaia
Goddess of the earth

Hera
Goddess of marriage

Nyx
Goddess of the night

Phoebe
Goddess of intellect

Rhea
Goddess of fertility

Theia
Goddess of sight

Thesis
Goddess of creation

Gods (Greek)

Adonis
God of beauty and desire

Atlas
God of astronomy

Dionysus
God of wine

Epimetheus
God of afterthought

Eros
God of love

Hermes
Messenger of the gods

Hyperion
God of light

Poseidon
God of the sea

Prometheus
God of forethought

Zeus
King of the gods

Goddesses (Roman)

Annona
Goddess of grain

Ceres
Goddess of fertility and the harvest

Flora
Goddess of flowers

Juno
Queen of the gods

Luna
Goddess of the moon

Maia
Goddess of growth

Minerva
Goddess of wisdom

Proserpina
Goddess of the underworld

Venus
Goddess of love

Vesta
Goddess of the home

Gods (Roman)

Apollo
God of the sun

Bacchus
God of wine

Cupid
God of love

Janus
God of doorways and gateways

Jupiter
God of sky and thunder

Mars
God of war

Mercury
Messenger of the gods

Neptune
God of the sea

Plutus
God of wealth

Vulcan
God of fire and smithery

Golfers

Annika Sörenstam
Born 1970, successful Swedish golfer

Babe Didrikson Zaharias
1911–1956, multi-talented American athlete

Betsy King
Born 1955, American, major championship winner

Karrie Webb
Born 1974, top Australian golfer

Laura Davies
Born 1963, most accomplished female British player

Mickey Wright
Born 1935, American, World Golf Hall of Fame member

Patty Berg
1918–2006, American, founding member of the LPGA Tour

Sun-Ju Ahn
Born 1987, South Korean tour winner

Suzann Pettersen
Born 1981, Norwegian, LPGA tour and major winner

Yani Tseng
Born 1989, Taiwanese, youngest player to win five majors

Golfers

Arnold Palmer
Born 1929, American golf legend

Byron Nelson
1912–2006, top American player

Ernie Els
Born 1969, South African golf star

Francis Ouimet
1893–1967, American 'father of amateur golf'

Greg Norman
Born 1955, Australian former world number one

Jack Nicklaus
Born 1940, American icon, aka 'The Golden Bear'

Nick Faldo
Born 1957, English, six-time major winner

Seve Ballesteros
1957–2011, Spanish, former world number one

Tiger Woods
Born 1975, American, top-earning golfer of all time

Walter Hagen
1892–1969, American, multiple major championship winner

Guitarists

Ani DiFranco
Born 1970, American musician, singer-songwriter and feminist icon

Bonnie Raitt
Born 1949, American blues writer and performer

Carrie Brownstein
Born 1974, American frontwoman of Sleater-Kinney

Janis Ian
Born 1951, legendary American musician

Joni Mitchell
Born 1943, influential Canadian singer-songwriter

Kaki King
Born 1979, American guitarist and composer

Lita Ford
Born 1958, British-born American, Runaways guitarist

Marnie Stern
Born 1976, American songwriter and technically gifted guitarist

Maybelle Carter
1909–1978, American country musician, member of the Carter Family

Wanda Jackson
Born 1937, American 'first lady of rockabilly'

Guitarists

Bo Diddley
1928–2008, influential American rock 'n' roll performer

Carlos Santana
Born 1947, Mexican–American guitar legend

Clarence White
1944–1973, Canadian–American guitarist with The Byrds

Django Reinhardt
1910–1953, virtuoso jazz guitar pioneer

Eddie Van Halen
Born 1955, Dutch–American frontman and co-founder of Van Halen

Eric Clapton
Born 1945, decorated English guitar legend

Jimi Hendrix
1942–1970, American electric guitar god

Kurt Cobain
1967–1994, American frontman of Nirvana

Link Wray
1929–2005, American rock 'n' roll guitarist and songwriter

Thurston Moore
Born 1958, American frontman of Sonic Youth

Historians

Amanda Foreman
Born 1968, British–American biographer and historian

Anita Brookner
Born 1928, English novelist and art historian

Antonia Fraser
Born 1932, English biographer and novelist

Barbara Tuchman
1912–1989, American historian and author

Claire Andrieu
Born 1952, French political historian

Kathleen Kenyon
1906–1978, English historian and archaeologist

Marjorie Rosen
Born 1942, American journalist, screenwriter and historian

Mary Ritter Beard
1876–1958, American historian and archivist

Meridel Le Sueur
1900–1996, American writer and historian

Ursula Hoff
1909–2005, Australian writer and art historian

Historians

Bartolomé de las Casas
1484–1566, Spanish historian, explorer and politician

Carter Godwin Woodson
1875–1950, African-American historian and journalist

Domingo Faustino Sarmiento
1811–1888, Argentinian president and historian

Eric Hobsbawm
1917–2012, British Marxist historian

Ernst Gombrich
1909–2001, Austrian-born British art historian

Fernand Braudel
1902–1985, French historian and teacher

Leonard Dupee White
1891–1958, American public administration historian

Max Hastings
Born 1945, English historian and journalist

Quentin Skinner
Born 1940, English historian and teacher

Simon Schama
Born 1945, English historian and professor

Illustrators

Barbara Bradley
1927–2008, pioneering American illustrator

Dyna Moe
Born 1978, American *Mad Men* illustrator

Janet Ahlberg
1944–1994, English children's book illustrator

Jessie Willcox Smith
1863–1935, American children's book and magazine illustrator

Kate Greenaway
1846–1901, English children's illustrator and writer

Marilyn Conover
Born 1926, American magazine illustrator

Olive Rush
1873–1966, American illustrator and muralist

Tove Jansson
1914–2001, Finnish creator of the Moomins

Trina Schart Hyman
1939–2004, American children's book illustrator

Violet Oakley
1874–1961, American illustrator and muralist

Illustrators

Arthur Rackham
1867–1939, English book illustrator

Axel Scheffler
Born 1957, German illustrator of *The Gruffalo*

Coby Whitmore
1913–1988, American magazine illustrator

Edmund Dulac
1882–1953, French book illustrator

Maurice Sendak
1928–2012, American creator of *Where the Wild Things Are*

Newell Convers Wyeth
1882–1945, American book and magazine illustrator

Kay Nielsen
1886–1957, Danish Art Nouveau illustrator

Quentin Blake
Born 1932, English illustrator of Roald Dahl's books

Simms Taback
1932–2011, award-winning American illustrator

Theodor Geisel (Dr Seuss)
1904–1991, legendary American children's book creator

Inventors

Bette Nesmith Graham
1924–1980, American inventor of correction fluid

Giuliana Tesoro
1921–2002, prolific Italian–American inventor, holding over 125 patents

Josephine Garis Cochrane
1839–1913, American, created the first mechanical dishwasher

Margaret Knight
1838–1914, prolific American inventor, aka 'the female Edison'

Marion Donovan
1917–1998, American who developed first disposable 'diaper'

Mary Phelps Jacob
1891–1970, American inventor of the modern bra

Melitta Bentz
1873–1950, German inventor of the coffee filter

Stephanie Kwolek
Born 1923, Polish–American chemist and inventor

Temple Grandin
Born 1947, autistic American inventor and activist

Virginia Apgar
1909–1974, developed the Apgar score to assess the health of newborn babies

Inventors

Alexander Graham Bell
1847–1922, Scottish inventor of the telephone

Barthélemy Thimonnier
1793–1857, French inventor of the sewing machine

Christopher Latham Sholes
1819–1890, American inventor of the typewriter

Eli Whitney
1765–1825, American inventor of the cotton gin

George de Mestral
1907–1990, Swiss inventor of Velcro

Gottlieb Daimler
1834–1900, German inventor of the four-wheel car

Hubert Cecil Booth
1871–1955, English inventor of the vacuum cleaner

Percy Spencer
1894–1970, American inventor of the microwave oven

Thomas Edison
1847–1931, American, one of the world's most prolific inventors

Tim Berners-Lee
Born 1955, English inventor of the World Wide Web

Journalists

Allegra Stratton
Born 1980, English, political editor of *Newsnight*

Arianna Huffington
Born 1950, American co-founder of *The Huffington Post*

Ayala Hasson-Nesher
Born 1961, Israeli journalist and TV personality

Decca Aitkenhead
Born 1971, English award-winning *Guardian* journalist

Eileen Welsome
Born 1951, American Pulitzer Prize winner

Gloria Steinem
Born 1934, American co-founder of *Ms.* magazine

Jane Hamsher
Born 1959, American film producer, activist and journalist

Katharine Whitehorn
Born 1928, British feminist journalist

Marie Colvin
1956–2012, American award-winning *Sunday Times* journalist

Pearl Stewart
Born 1950, African-American newspaper editor

Journalists

Carl Bernstein
Born 1944, American, uncovered Watergate scandal

Elijah Parish Lovejoy
1802–1837, American voice against slavery

Elmer Davis
1890–1958, American news reporter and recipient of the Peabody Award

Hunter S. Thompson
1937–2005, American instigator of 'gonzo' (subjective) journalism

John Zenger
1697–1746, German–American advocate of press freedom

Joseph Pulitzer
1847–1911, Hungarian–American, father of modern journalism

Paul Foot
1937–2004, British investigative journalist and political campaigner

Robert Fisk
Born 1946, English, Middle East correspondent for the *Independent*

Seymour Hersh
Born 1937, award-winning American investigative journalist

Wilfred Burchett
1911–1983, Australian war journalist

Lawyers

Bella Abzug
1920–1998, American congresswoman, activist and lawyer

Belva Lockwood
1830–1917, American lawyer, politician and activist

Brenda Hale
Born 1945, English, first woman to become a law lord

Charlotte Ray
1850–1911, African-American civil rights lawyer

Cherie Booth
Born 1954, top English barrister and QC

Elizabeth Edwards
1949–2010, American senator, author and lawyer

Geraldine Ferraro
1935–2011, American lawyer and congresswoman

Helena Kennedy
Born 1950, Scottish barrister and broadcaster

Michelle Obama
Born 1964, American lawyer and First Lady

Shirin Ebadi
Born 1947, Iranian Nobel Peace Prize winner

Lawyers

Alexander Hamilton
1755–1804, American Founding Father, born Nevis, West Indies

Barack Obama
Born 1961, American president, lawyer and author

Chester Arthur
1829–1886, American president and lawyer

Hugo Black
1886–1971, American Supreme Court justice

Francis Bacon
1561–1626, English lawyer, scientist and politician

Raúl Alfonsín
1927–2009, Argentinian president and lawyer

René Cassin
1887–1976, French lawyer and anti-war activist

Tony Blair
Born 1953, British prime minister and lawyer

Thurgood Marshall
1908–1993, African-American Supreme Court Justice

William Garrow
1760–1840, British barrister, judge and politician

Magicians

Adelaide Herrmann
1853–1932, English illusionist and vaudeville performer

Ava Do
Born 1979, Vietnamese magician and writer

Billy Kid
Born 1982, Canadian magician and street performer

Celeste Evans
Born 1931, Canadian specialising in dove magic

Dell O'Dell
1902–1962, pioneering American magician and juggler

Kleo Dorotti
1900–1974, Russian illusionist

Luna Shimada
Born 1966, Australian conjuror

Misty Lee
Born 1976, American magician and comedian

Okita
1852–1916, British linking rings specialist

Trixie Bond
Born 1955, American magician and inventor

Magicians

Dai Vernon
1894–1992, Canadian sleight-of-hand magician

Dante
1883–1955, Danish 'Golden Age' magician

David Copperfield
Born 1956, internationally famous American illusionist

Derren Brown
Born 1971, English illusionist and hypnotist

Doug Henning
1947–2000, Canadian escape artist

Harry Houdini
1874–1926, Hungarian–American stunt performer

Lance Burton
Born 1960, American, Las Vegas magician

Paul Daniels
Born 1938, Britain's favourite TV magician

Richiardi
1923–1985, Peruvian illusionist

Siegfried Fischbacher
Born 1939, German–American half of Siegfried & Roy

Mathematicians

Amalie Emmy Noether
1882–1935, German specialist in abstract algebra

Bhama Srinivasan
Born 1935, influential Indian mathematician

Florence Allen
1876–1960, pioneering American mathematician

Gabrielle Émilie le Tonnelier de Breteuil
1706–1749, French mathematician and scientific author

Julia Hall Bowman Robinson
1919–1985, influential American mathematician

Maria Gaetana Agnesi
1718–1799, Italian mathematician and philosopher

Marie–Sophie Germain
1776–1831, French theory and geometry specialist

Mary Lucy Cartwright
1900–1998, English, focused on function theory

Sofia Vasilyevna Kovalevskaya
1850–1891, Russian mathematician and teacher

Sun–Yung Alice Chang
Born 1948, Chinese–American mathematician and professor

Mathematicians

Carl Gauss
1777–1855, German mathematician and physical scientist

Euclid
c.300 BC, Greek 'father of geometry'

Fibonacci
c.1170–c.1250, influential Italian mathematician

Georg Cantor
1845–1918, German inventor of set theory

Girolamo Cardano
1501–1576, Italian Renaissance mathematician

Grigori Perelman
Born 1966, landmark Russian mathematician

John Horton Conway
Born 1937, English recreational mathematician

Leonhard Euler
1707–1783, influential Swiss mathematician, dubbed 'analysis incarnate'

Pythagoras
c.570 BC–c.495 BC, Greek mathematician famous for his theorem

Terry Tao
Born 1975, medal-winning Australian mathematician

Military Leaders

Agustina de Aragón
1786–1857, Spanish War of Independence heroine

Ahhotep I
c.1560 BC–c.1530 BC, Egyptian queen and defender of Thebes

Artemisia I of Caria
c.480 BC, queen and naval commander of Ionia

Boudica
Died c.60, British queen of Iceni tribe, led uprising against the Romans

Fu Hao
Died c.1200 BC, Chinese military general and high priestess

Joan of Arc
1412–1431, French, led army in Hundred Years' War

Tamar of Georgia
1160–1213, Georgian ruler and warrior

Triệu Thị Trinh
AD 225–248, led Vietnamese rebellion against Chinese rule

Tomoe Gozen
c.1157–1247, Japanese samurai warrior

Zenobia
AD 240–274, Syrian queen, led revolt against Roman Empire

Military Leaders

Alexander the Great
356 BC–323 BC, Macedonian, conquered much of known world

Charlemagne
AD 742–814, German founder of Carolingian Empire

Che Guevara
1928–1967, Argentinian guerrilla leader, real name 'Ernesto'

Cyrus the Great
c.600 BC–c.530 BC, founder of Archaemendid Persian Empire

Genghis Khan
1162–1227, Mongolian, founder and iron ruler of the vast Mongol Empire

Hannibal
247 BC–c.183 BC, Carthaginian military commander

Horatio Nelson
1758–1805, English naval commander during Napoleonic Wars

Napoleon Bonaparte
1769–1821, French general and self-appointed First Consul

Richard I
1157–1199, English king, led the Third Crusade, aka Richard the Lionheart

Saladin
1138–1193, Kurdish, led Muslim opposition to European crusades

Monarchs (Ancient)

Ankhesenamun
*c.*1348 BC–*c.*1322 BC, queen of Egypt

Arsinoë II
*c.*316 BC–*c.*270 BC, queen of Thrace, Asia Minor and Macedonia

Cleopatra VII
69–30 BC, the last pharaoh of Ancient Egypt

Hatshepsut
*c.*1508–*c.*1458 BC, Ancient Egyptian, longest-reigning female pharaoh

Helena
*c.*246–*c.*330, Roman empress, mother of Constantine

Livia Drusilla
58 BC–AD 29, Roman empress, wife and adviser to Augustus Caesar

Nefertiti
*c.*1370 BC–*c.*1330 BC, Egyptian 'Lady of Grace'

Olympias
*c.*375 BC–316 BC, Greek princess, ruler and mother of Alexander the Great

Shammuramat
Ninth century BC, queen of Assyria and basis for the legends of Semiramis

Tomyris
*c.*530 BC, queen of Persia

Monarchs (Ancient)

Alfred the Great
849–899, Anglo-Saxon king of Wessex

Canute
985–1035, king of Denmark, England and Norway

Darius I
c.550–c.486 BC, king of Persia

Ethelred the Unready
968–1016, twice king of England

Haakon Sigurdsson
c.937–995, king of Norway

Pepi II
c.2278 BC–c.2184 BC, Ancient Egyptian pharaoh

Sweyn Forkbeard
c.960–1014, king of Denmark and England

Tiberius
42 BC–AD 37, Roman emperor

Tutankhamun
c.1341–1323 BC, most well-known Egyptian pharaoh

Xerxes II
Died 424 BC, Persian king, assassinated by his brother

Monarchs (Modern)

Beatrix
Born 1938, queen of the Netherlands

Catherine the Great
1729–1796, empress of Russia

Elizabeth II
Born 1926, queen of England and head of the Commonwealth

Henrietta Maria of France
1609–1669, queen consort of England

Juliana
1909–2004, queen of the Netherlands

Margrethe II
Born 1940, queen of Denmark

Mary II
1662–1694, co-ruler of England with William III

Nur Jahan
1577–1645, empress of Mughal Empire, for whom the Taj Mahal was built

Sophia of Hanover
1630–1714, German electress, narrowly missed out on English throne

Ulrika Eleanora
1688–1741, queen of Sweden

Monarchs (Modern)

Abdullah II
Born 1962, king of Jordan

Akihito
Born 1933, emperor of Japan

Albert II
Born 1934, king of Belgium

Charles I
1600–1649, king of England

Harald V
Born 1937, king of Norway

Isa ibn Ali Al Khalifa
1848–1932, king of Bahrain

Jigme Khesar Namgyel Wangchuck
Born 1980, Dragon King of Kingdom of Bhutan

Letsie III
Born 1963, king of Lesotho

Norodom Sihamoni
Born 1953, king of Cambodia

Oscar I
1799–1859, king of Sweden and Norway

Mountaineers

Alison Hargreaves
1963–1995, English adventurer, scaled Everest solo

Anna Czerwińska
Born 1949, Polish, oldest woman to summit Everest

Arlene Blum
Born 1945, American mountaineer and environmentalist

Edurne Pasaban
Born 1973, Basque Spanish mountaineer

Eylem Elif Mavis
Born 1973, first Turkish woman to climb Everest

Ginette Harrison
1958–1999, English, first woman to summit Kangchenjunga

Isabella Bird
1831–1904, British explorer and natural historian

Junko Tabei
Born 1939, Japanese climber, first woman to summit Everest

Meta Brevoort
1825–1876, American, first woman to climb the Matterhorn

Phyllis Munday
1894–1990, Canadian mountaineer and naturalist

Mountaineers

Albert Mummery
1855–1895, much-respected English mountaineer

Clinton Thomas Dent
1850–1912, English surgeon, writer and alpinist

Darby Field
1610–1649, Irish, first European to climb Mount Washington in New Hampshire

Dean Potter
Born 1972, American BASE jumper and free climber

Edmund Hillary
1919–2008, New Zealand climber, first to summit Everest (with Tenzing Norgay)

Jesse Guthrie
Born 1958, pioneering American sport climber

Kenton Cool
Born 1973, a leading British alpine climber

Reinhold Messner
Born 1944, German–Italian, considered greatest climber in history

Tenzing Norgay
1914–1986, Nepali mountaineer, first to summit Everest (with Edmund Hillary)

Walter Bonatti
1930–2011, Italian climber, first solo winter ascent of Matterhorn north face

Olympians (Summer)

Alice Coachman
Born 1923, American high jumper

Dawn Fraser
Born 1937, Australian swimmer

Florence Griffith Joyner
1959–1998, American sprinter

Jessica Ennis
Born 1986, English heptathlete

Katherine Grainger
Born 1975, Scottish rower

Wu Minxia
Born 1985, Chinese diver

Misty May-Treanor
Born 1977, American beach volleyball player

Nadia Comaneci
Born 1961, Romanian gymnast

Valentina Vezzali
Born 1974, Italian fencer

Victoria Pendleton
Born 1980, English track cyclist

Olympians (Summer)

Bradley Wiggins
Born 1980, English track and road cyclist

Emil Zátopek
1922–2000, Czech long-distance runner

Jesse Owens
1913–1980, American sprinter and long jumper

Kenenisa Bekele
Born 1982, Ethiopian long-distance runner

Linford Christie
Born 1960, Jamaican-born British sprinter

Michael Phelps
Born 1985, American swimmer

Mo Farah
Born 1983, Somali-born British distance runner

Paavo Nurmi
1897–1973, Finnish long-distance runner

Usain Bolt
Born 1986, Jamaican sprinter

Viktor Saneyev
Born 1945, Russian triple jumper

Olympians (Winter)

Chemmy Alcott
Born 1982, British champion skier

Christa Luding-Rothenburger
Born 1959, German speed skater

Clara Hughes
Born 1972, Canadian speed skater

Claudia Pechstein
Born 1972, German speed skater

Jayne Torvill
Born 1957, English ice dancer

Larissa Lazutina
Born 1965, Russian cross-country skier

Lidiya Skoblikova
Born 1939, Russian speed skater

Marja-Liisa Hämäläinen
Born 1955, Finnish cross-country skier

Raisa Smetanina
Born 1952, Russian cross-country skier

Sonja Henie
1912–1969, Norwegian figure skater

Olympians (Winter)

Alberto Tomba
Born 1966, Italian slalom skier

Bjorn Daehlie
Born 1967, Norwegian cross-country skier

Eugenio Monti
1928–2003, Italian bobsledder

Felix Loch
Born 1989, German luger and Olympic champion

Gillis Grafström
1893–1938, Swedish figure skater and Olympic champion

Joji Kato
Born 1985, Japanese speed skater

Masahiko Harada
Born 1968, Japanese ski jumper

Ole Einar Bjorndalen
Born 1974, Norwegian biathlete

Robel Teklemariam
Born 1974, Ethiopian cross-country skier

Vladislav Tretiak
Born 1952, Russian ice hockey player

Paralympians

Chantal Benoit
Born 1960, Canadian wheelchair basketball player

Yu Chui Yee
Born 1984, Chinese wheelchair fencer

Ellie Simmonds
Born 1994, English swimmer

Esther Vergeer
Born 1981, Dutch wheelchair tennis player

Hannah Cockroft
Born 1992, English wheelchair athlete

Helene Raynsford
Born 1979, English rower

Karissa Whitsell
Born 1981, American blind cyclist

Paola Fantato
Born 1959, Italian archer

Tanni Grey-Thompson
Born 1969, Welsh wheelchair racer

Viviane Forest
Born 1979, Canadian goalball player and skier

Paralympians

Antonio Tenório da Silva
Born 1970, Brazilian judoka

David Weir
Born 1979, Scottish wheelchair racer

Jiri Jezek
Born 1974, Czech road and track cyclist

Jonas Jacobsson
Born 1965, Swedish shooter

Jonnie Peacock
Born 1993, English sprinter

Oscar Pistorius
Born 1986, South African sprinter

Pál Szekeres
Born 1964, Hungarian fencer

Richard Whitehead
Born 1976, English track athlete

Troy Sachs
Born 1975, Australian wheelchair basketball player

Volodymyr Antonyuk
Born 1972, Ukrainian footballer

Philosophers

Antoinette Bourignon
1616–1680, Belgian religious philosopher

Ayn Rand
1905–1982, Russian–American philosopher and best-selling author

Julia Domna
AD 170–217, Roman empress and philosopher

Margaret Cavendish
1623–1673, English philosopher, writer and scientist

Marie de Gournay
1565–1645, French feminist philosopher

Nancy Cartwright
Born 1944, American professor of philosophy

Philippa Foot
1920–2010, English founder of virtue ethics

Rosalind Hursthouse
Born 1943, New Zealand moral philosopher

Simone de Beauvoir
1908–1986, French existentialist philosopher

Themistoclea
Sixth century BC, Ancient Greek philosopher and priestess

Philosophers

Aristotle
384–322 BC, Ancient Greek 'godfather of philosophy'

Auguste Comte
1798–1857, French founder of sociology

Bertrand Russell
1872–1970, British founder of analytical philosophy

Friedrich Nietzsche
1844–1900, radical German philosopher

Georg Hegel
1770–1831, German idealist philosopher

Immanuel Kant
1724–1804, German philosopher, coined term 'Enlightenment'

Ludwig Wittgenstein
1889–1951, Austrian–British philosopher fascinated with language

Martin Heidegger
1889–1976, German existential philosopher

René Descartes
1596–1650, French 'father of modern philosophy'

Soren Kierkegaard
1813–1855, Danish 'father of existentialism'

Photographers

Annie Liebovitz
Born 1949, American magazine portrait photographer

Camille Silvy
1834–1910, French pioneer of early photography

Cindy Sherman
Born 1954, American self-portraitist

Corinne Day
1965–2010, English fashion photographer

Diane Arbus
1923–1971, American portrait photographer of alternative society

Helen Levitt
1913–2009, American street photographer

Julia Margaret Cameron
1815–1879, British portrait pioneer

Nan Goldin
Born 1953, controversial American photographer

Polly Borland
Born 1959, Australian portrait photographer

Rollie McKenna
1918–2003, American portraitist

Photographers

Ansel Adams
1902–1984, American wilderness landscape photographer

Arthur Fellig
1899–1968, Austrian–American crime scene photographer, aka 'Weegee'

David Bailey
Born 1938, English photography legend

Emil Otto Hoppé
1878–1972, German-born British travel and portrait photographer

Henri Cartier-Bresson
1908–2004, French black-and-white master

Irving Penn
1917–2009, American portraitist and fashion photographer

Mario Testino
Born 1954, Peruvian fashion photographer

Philippe Halsman
1906–1979, Latvian–American portrait photographer

Richard Avedon
1923–2004, American 'father of modern photography'

Walker Evans
1903–1975, American street photographer

Physicists

Chien-Shiung Wu
1912–1997, Chinese-born American expert in radioactivity

Émilie du Châtelet
1706–1749, French physicist, mathematician and author

Inge Lehmann
1888–1993, Danish seismologist

Jocelyn Bell Burnell
Born 1943, Northern Irish astrophysicist

Lene Hau
Born 1959, award-winning Danish physicist

Lisa Randall
Born 1962, American theoretical physicist and cosmologist

Lise Meitner
1878–1968, Austrian–Swedish nuclear physicist

Marie Curie
1867–1934, French–Polish Nobel Prize-winning physicist, discovered radium

Rosalind Franklin
1920–1958, English biophysicist and X-ray crystallographer

Shirley Ann Jackson
Born 1946, American nuclear physicist

Physicists

Albert Einstein
1879–1955, German-born genius, developed theory of relativity

Benjamin Franklin
1706–1790, American polymath, helped discover electricity

Brian Cox
Born 1968, English particle physicist and TV presenter

Enrico Fermi
1901–1954, Italian-born, helped develop first nuclear reactor

Erwin Schrödinger
1887–1961, Austrian, revolutionised quantum mechanics

Isaac Newton
1642–1727, English physicist, described gravitation and the three laws of motion

Max Planck
1858–1947, German Nobel Prize-winning originator of quantum theory

Michael Faraday
1791–1867, English electromagnetism and electrochemistry pioneer

Nikola Tesla
1856–1943, Serbian–American theoretical physicist, inventor and engineer

Stephen Hawking
Born 1942, English theoretical physicist and author

Pianists

Clara Schumann
1819–1896, German Romantic pianist

Diana Krall
Born 1964, Canadian jazz pianist and singer

Fiona Apple
Born 1977, American pianist and singer-songwriter

Ilona Eibenschütz
1872–1967, Hungarian concert pianist

Marcelle Meyer
1897–1958, influential French pianist

Moura Lympany
1916–2005, English concert pianist

Myra Hess
1890–1965, English pianist

Regina Spektor
Born 1980, American singer-songwriter and pianist

Rosa Tamarkina
1920–1950, prize-winning Russian pianist

Tarja Turunen
Born 1977, Finnish pianist and singer-songwriter

Pianists

Aaron Goldberg
Born 1974, American jazz pianist

Alfred Cortot
1877–1962, Swiss–French pianist, professor and conductor

Arthur Rubinstein
1887–1982, successful Polish–American pianist

Emil Gilels
1916–1985, Russian concert pianist

Glenn Gould
1932–1982, celebrated eccentric Canadian pianist

Jamie Cullum
Born 1979, English jazz-pop pianist and singer

Sergei Rachmaninov
1873–1943, legendary Russian pianist and composer

Sviatoslav Richter
1915–1997, Russian virtuoso pianist

Vladimir Horowitz
1903–1989, legendary Russian–American pianist

Wilhelm Kempff
1895–1991, German pianist and composer

Playwrights

Aphra Behn
1640–1689, English dramatist of the Restoration period

Augusta Gregory
1852–1932, founder of the Irish Literary Theatre

Delarivier Manley
c.1670–1724, English playwright and political pamphleteer

Hattie Gossett
Born 1942, African-American feminist playwright

Joanna Baillie
1762–1851, prolific Scottish playwright

Mary Zimmerman
Born 1960, American playwright and director

Nancy Oliver
Born 1955, American playwright and screenwriter

Pamela Gien
Born 1957, South African creator of *The Syringa Tree*

Polly Stenham
Born 1986, award-winning English playwright

Sharon Pollock
Born 1936, Canadian playwright and actor

Playwrights

Anton Chekhov
1860–1904, Russian dramatist, novelist and short-story writer

Arthur Miller
1915–2005, American Pulitzer Prize-winning playwright

Eugene O'Neill
1888–1953, American playwright and Nobel laureate

George Bernard Shaw
1856–1950, Irish playwright and novelist

Harold Pinter
1930–2008, Nobel Prize-winning English playwright

Henrik Ibsen
1828–1906, Norwegian playwright and poet

Noël Coward
1899–1973, English playwright and composer

Seán O'Casey
1880–1964, pioneering Irish playwright

Tom Stoppard
Born 1937, decorated British playwright and screenwriter

William Shakespeare
1564–1616, English, the greatest playwright of them all

Poets

Amy Lowell
1874–1925, American Pulitzer Prize winner

Anna Akhmatova
1889–1966, acclaimed Russian poet

Carol Ann Duffy
Born 1955, British poet laureate

Christina Rossetti
1830–1894, English Romantic and children's poet

Elizabeth Bishop
1911–1979, award-winning American poet

Emily Dickinson
1830–1886, reclusive American poet

Lynette Roberts
1909–1995, Argentinian-born British poet

Marina Tsvetaeva
1892–1941, exiled Russian poet

Sappho
c.630 BC–c.570 BC, Ancient Greek lyric poet

Sylvia Plath
1932–1963, American confessional poet

Poets

Dylan Thomas
1914–1953, Welsh poet and writer

John Keats
1795–1821, English Romantic poet

Philip Larkin
1922–1985, English poet and novelist

Seamus Heaney
Born 1939, Irish poet and playwright

Siegfried Sassoon
1886–1967, English World War One poet

Ted Hughes
1930–1998, British poet and children's writer

Walt Whitman
1819–1892, American poet and journalist

Wilfred Owen
1893–1918, English World War One poet

William Wordsworth
1770–1850, English Romantic poet

Wystan Hugh Auden
1907–1973, Anglo-American poet

Political Leaders

Angela Merkel
Born 1954, first female chancellor of Germany

Benazir Bhutto
1953–2007, twice Pakistani prime minister

Catherine the Great
1729–1796, longest-ruling female Russian leader

Ellen Johnson Sirleaf
Born 1938, Liberian president, first elected female head of state in Africa

Golda Meir
1898–1978, first female prime minister of Israel

Sheikh **Hasina** Wajed
Born 1947, Bangladeshi prime minister

Helle Thorning-Schmidt
Born 1966, Danish prime minister

Indira Ghandi
1917–1984, four-time prime minister of India

Jóhanna Sigurðardóttir
Born 1942, prime minister of Iceland

Julia Gillard
Born 1961, Australian prime minister

Political Leaders

Abraham Lincoln
1809–1865, American president who brought an end to slavery

Benjamin Disraeli
1804–1881, British prime minister and literary figure

Charles de Gaulle
1890–1970, French president and army general

Franklin Delano Roosevelt
1882–1945, American president during the Great Depression

George Washington
1732–1799, first American president

Harold Wilson
1916–1995, twice British prime minister

Julius Caesar
100–44 BC, Ancient Rome's famous leader

Nelson Mandela
Born 1918, South African president

Vladimir Lenin
1870–1924, Russian founder of the Soviet Union

Winston Churchill
1874–1965, British prime minister during World War Two

Psychologists

Anna Freud
1895–1982, Austrian psychoanalyst

Dorothea Dix
1802–1887, American, introduced psychiatric institutions

Florence Goodenough
1886–1959, American psychologist and professor

Karen Horney
1885–1952, German psychoanalyst

Leta Hollingworth
1886–1939, American educational psychologist

Mamie Phipps Clark
1917–1983, African-American social psychologist

Mary Calkins
1863–1930, American psychologist and philosopher

Melanie Klein
1882–1960, Austrian-born British psychoanalyst

Ruth Howard
1900–1997, African-American social psychologist

Sabina Spielrein
1885–1942, Russian psychoanalyst and physician

Psychologists

Albert Bandura
Born 1925, Canadian–American cognitive revolutionist

Alfred Adler
1870–1937, Austrian psychotherapist and medical doctor

Carl Jung
1875–1961, Swiss analytical psychologist

Erik Erikson
1902–1994, German-born American developmental psychologist

Gordon Allport
1897–1967, American personality psychologist

Ivan Pavlov
1849–1936, Russian animal behaviour psychologist and physiologist

Jean Piaget
1896–1980, Swiss children's psychologist

Kurt Lewin
1890–1947, German–American 'father of modern psychology'

Sigmund Freud
1856–1939, Austrian 'godfather of psychoanalysis'

Stanley Milgram
1933–1984, American social psychologist

Racing Drivers

Ana Beatriz de Figueiredo
Born 1985, Brazilian, first woman to win an Indy Lights Series race, aka Bia

Ashley Force Hood
Born 1982, American Funny Car drag racer

Danica Patrick
Born 1982, American, first woman to lead the Indy 500

Jennifer Jo Cobb
Born 1973, American NASCAR racing driver

Maria de Villota
Born 1980, Spanish, F1 test driver

Maryeve Dufault
Born 1982, Canadian–American racing driver and model

Milka Duno
Born 1972, Venezuelan IndyCar driver

Pippa Mann
Born 1983, English IndyCar driver

Simona de Silvestro
Born 1988, Swiss IndyCar driver

Susie Wolff
Born 1982, Scottish, F1 development driver

Racing Drivers

Alain Prost
Born 1955, French four-time F1 world champion

Ayrton Senna
1960–1994, Brazilian three-time F1 world champion

Damon Hill
Born 1960, English F1 world champion driver

Fernando Alonso
Born 1981, Spanish, twice F1 world champion

Jacques Villeneuve
Born 1971, multi-championship-winning Canadian F1 driver

Jenson Button
Born 1980, English F1 world champion

Lewis Hamilton
Born 1985, English F1 world champion

Michael Schumacher
Born 1969, German seven-time F1 world champion

Sebastian Vettel
Born 1987, German F1 world champion

Stirling Moss
Born 1929, legendary British F1 racing driver

Radio Personalities

Annie Nightingale
Born 1940, English, longest-serving presenter on BBC Radio 1

Carolina Bermudez
Born 1978, American radio DJ

Devon Angelica
Born 1985, American radio and TV presenter

Kirsty Young
Born 1968, Scottish presenter of *Desert Island Discs*

Lauren Laverne
Born 1978, English radio DJ and TV personality

Liz Wilde
Born 1971, American radio 'shock jock'

Louise Elliott
Born 1969, Welsh radio and TV presenter

Marjorie Anderson
1913–1999, English long-running presenter of *Woman's Hour*

Martha Kearney
Born 1957, Irish radio news presenter

Nemone Metaxas
Born 1973, English BBC radio DJ and TV presenter

Radio Personalities

Alastair Cooke
1908–2004, British–American radio and TV presenter

Aled Jones
Born 1970, Welsh singer and radio and TV presenter

Arthur Askey
1900–1982, English comedian and radio personality

Christopher Stone
1882–1965, Britain's first radio DJ

Howard Stern
Born 1954, outspoken American radio DJ

John Peel
1939–2004, legendary English radio presenter

Reginald Fessenden
1866–1932, Canadian–American, transmitted first radio broadcast

Tony Blackburn
Born 1943, English, first DJ to broadcast on BBC Radio 1

Walter Winchell
1897–1972, American radio presenter, coined term 'disc jockey'

Zane Lowe
Born 1973, New Zealand DJ, record producer and TV presenter

Rappers

Deidra Roper
Born 1971, American, member of Salt-N-Pepa, aka 'DJ Spinderella'

Eve
Born 1978, American Grammy-winning rapper, songwriter and record producer

Foxy Brown
Born 1978, American rap soloist and collaborator

Jacki-O
Born 1975, Haitian–American rapper and actor

Lauryn Hill
Born 1975, American, one-time Fugees frontwoman

Lisa Left Eye Lopes
1971–2002, American, one-third of TLC

Missy Elliott
Born 1971, American rap legend

Monie Love
Born 1970, English performer

Nicki Minaj
Born 1984, Trinidadian–American rapper and voice actor

Trina
Born 1978, American rapper and model

Rappers

André 3000
Born 1975, American member of OutKast

Chuck D
Born 1960, American rapper and producer

Jay-Z
Born 1969, multi-award winning American performer

Kanye West
Born 1977, American musician and fashion designer

Marshall Mathers
Born 1972, American, aka 'Eminem'

Nas
Born 1973, successful American rapper and actor

Raekwon
Born 1970, American, member of the Wu-Tang Clan

Rakim
Born 1968, influential American performer

Tinchy Stryder
Born 1986, British hip hop performer

Tupac
1971–1996, African-American rap legend

Religious Leaders

Agnes Sigurðardóttir
Born 1954, Bishop of Iceland

Hildegard of Bingen
1098–1179, German Benedictine abbess

Ingrid Mattson
Born 1963, Canadian Islamic professor

Mary Baker Eddy
1821–1910, American founder of Christian Science

Mata Amritanandamayi
Born 1953, Indian Hindu spiritual leader

Penny Jamieson
Born 1942, New Zealand bishop

Sharon Kleinbaum
Born 1959, American rabbi and human and gay rights activist

Teresa of Calcutta (Mother Teresa)
1910–1997, Albanian-born missionary and charity worker

Veronica Giuliani
1660–1727, Italian Capuchin abbess

Yolanda of Poland
1235–1298, Hungarian abbess

Religious Leaders

Clement VII
1478–1534, Italian Medici pope

Desmond Tutu
Born 1931, South African human rights activist and Anglican bishop

Francis of Assisi
1181–1226, Italian Catholic friar and preacher, founder of the Franciscan order

Siddhārtha Gautama Buddha
c.563–c.483 BC, born in present-day Nepal; spiritual teachings led to Buddhism

Ignatius of Loyola
1491–1556, Spanish founder of the Jesuits

Jesus Christ
c.7 BC–AD 36, born in Roman-occupied Judaea, central figure of Christianity

Joseph Smith Jr
1805–1844, American founder of the Latter Day Saint movement

Muhammad
c.571–632, born in Arabia (Mecca); the prophet of Islam

Swami Sathyananda Saraswathi
1935–2006, Indian Hindu spiritual teacher

Tenzin Gyatso
Born 1935, Tibetan Dalai Lama

Rugby Players

Aida Ba
Born 1983, French flanker

Amber Penrith
Born 1980, England winger

Anaïs Lagougine
Born 1981, French winger

Cebisa Kula
Born 1981, South African prop

Emily Scarratt
Born 1990, England centre

Iliseva Batibasaga
Born 1985, Australian scrum half

Monalisa Codling
Born 1977, New Zealand lock

Phaidra Knight
Born 1974, American rugby icon

Rosemary Crowley
Born 1987, England prop

Sara Akerman
Born 1980, Swedish hooker

Rugby Players

Brian O'Driscoll
Born 1979, Irish captain

Buck Shelford
Born 1957, New Zealand player and coach

Gareth Edwards
Born 1947, Welsh scrum half

Hugo Porta
Born 1951, Argentinian fly half

Jonah Lomu
Born 1975, New Zealand winger

Jonny Wilkinson
Born 1979, England fly half and goal kicker

Martin Johnson
Born 1970, England player, captain and manager

Philippe Sella
Born 1962, record-breaking French centre

Serge Blanco
Born 1958, Venezuelan-born French fullback

Zinzan Brooke
Born 1965, New Zealand lock

Shakespearean Characters

Beatrice
Feisty heroine in *Much Ado About Nothing*

Cordelia
King Lear's brave and honest daughter

Helena
Brave gentlewoman in *All's Well That Ends Well*

Hermia
Romantic heroine of *A Midsummer Night's Dream*

Hero
Half of *Much Ado About Nothing*'s infatuated couple

Juliet
One half of star-crossed lovers *Romeo and Juliet*

Miranda
Young innocent in *The Tempest*

Portia
Determined heroine of *The Merchant of Venice*

Silvia
Lover of Valentine in *The Two Gentlemen of Verona*

Viola
Passionate heroine of *Twelfth Night*

Shakespearean Characters

Antonio
Melancholic protagonist of *The Merchant of Venice*

Demetrius
Young lover infatuated with Helena in *A Midsummer Night's Dream*

Duncan
Macbeth's king of Scotland

Falstaff
Supporting character who later earned a play of his own

Ferdinand
Earnest son of king Alonso in *The Tempest*

Hamlet
Tormented protagonist of eponymous play

Lysander
Hopeless romantic of *A Midsummer Night's Dream*

Malvolio
Dour servant in comedic *Twelfth Night*

Romeo
One half of tragic couple *Romeo and Juliet*

Tybalt
Capulet antagonist in *Romeo and Juliet*

Singers (Jazz)

Billie Holiday
1915–1959, American seminal jazz singer

Blossom Dearie
1924–2009, American jazz singer and pianist

Cleo Laine
Born 1927, English jazz singer known for her vocal range

Dee Dee Bridgewater
Born 1950, American Grammy and Tony winner

Ella Fitzgerald
1917–1996, American 'Queen of Jazz'

Ernestine Anderson
Born 1928, American jazz and blues performer

Nina Simone
1933–2003, American musical legend

Peggy Lee
1920–2002, American jazz and pop singer and actor

Reine Rimón
Born 1942, Finnish New Orleans jazz performer

Yaala Ballin
Born 1981, Israeli jazz vocalist and teacher

Singers (Jazz)

Alwin Jarreau
Born 1940, American multiple Grammy winner

Chet Baker
1929–1988, American jazz singer and trumpeter

Frank Sinatra
1915–1998, American musical superstar

Freddy Cole
Born 1931, American jazz singer and pianist

Louis Armstrong
1901–1971, American jazz trumpeter and singer, aka 'Satchmo'

Mel Tormé
1925–1999, American singer, composer and drummer, aka 'The Velvet Fog'

Nat King Cole
1919–1965, legendary American singer and pianist

Ola Onabule
Born 1964, British–Nigerian jazz and soul singer-songwriter, musician and producer

Ray Charles
1930–2004, American all-round legend

Vince Jones
Born 1954, Australian singer, songwriter and trumpet and flugelhorn player

Singers (Opera)

Carmen Monarcha
Born 1979, Brazilian soprano

Elisabeth Schwarzkopf
1915–2006, Austrian–British soprano

Grace Bumbry
Born 1937, American, mezzo-soprano

Joan Sutherland
1926–2010, Australian dramatic coloratura soprano

Kirsten Flagstad
1895–1962, Norwegian Wagnerian soprano

Lesley Garrett
Born 1955, English soprano and broadcaster

Maria Callas
1923–1977, American–Greek iconic soprano

Montserrat Caballé
Born 1933, Spanish soprano noted for her bel canto repertoire

Renata Tebaldi
1922–2004, Italian lirico-spinto soprano

Sissel Kyrkjebø
Born 1969, Norwegian crossover soprano

Singers (Opera)

Alfie Boe
Born 1973, English tenor

Andrea Bocelli
Born 1958, Italian crossover tenor

Dietrich Fischer-Dieskau
1925–2012, German lyric baritone and conductor

Dmitri Hvorostovsky
Born 1962, Russian baritone

José Carreras
Born 1946, Spanish–Catalan, one of 'The Three Tenors'

Jussi Björling
1911–1960, Swedish operatic tenor

Justino Díaz
Born 1940, Puerto Rican bass-baritone

Luciano Pavarotti
1935–2007, Italian, one of 'The Three Tenors'

Mario Lanza
1921–1959, American tenor and Hollywood star

Plácido Domingo
Born 1941, Spanish tenor and conductor, one of 'The Three Tenors'

Singers (Pop)

Adele Adkins
Born 1988, highly acclaimed English singer-songwriter

Barbra Streisand
Born 1942, American singer, actor, director and producer

Beyoncé Knowles
Born 1981, Grammy-winning American performer

Britney Spears
Born 1981, headline-grabbing American singer

Donna Summer
1948–2012, American star of disco era

Dusty Springfield
1939–1999, influential English performer

Madonna Ciccone
Born 1958, award-winning American artist

Pixie Lott
Born 1991, English singer-songwriter

Stevie Nicks
Born 1948, American singer-songwriter and vocalist with Fleetwood Mac

Whitney Houston
1963–2012, American singer and actor

Singers (Pop)

Barry Manilow
Born 1943, American pop favourite

Del Shannon
1934–1990, American singer-songwriter and guitarist

Ed Sheeran
Born 1991, English singer-songwriter and guitarist

Elton John
Born 1947, English singer, composer and pianist

John Lennon
1940–1980, English singer-songwriter and musician, member of the 'Fab Four'

Michael Jackson
1958–2009, American 'King of Pop'

Paul Simon
Born 1941, award-winning American musician and one half of Simon & Garfunkel

Phil Collins
Born 1951, English singer-songwriter, drummer and actor

Prince (Nelson)
Born 1958, Grammy-winning American singer-songwriter and musician

Rod Stewart
Born 1945, legendary British singer and musician

Singers (Rock)

Alanis Morissette
Born 1974, Canadian, Grammy-winning singer-songwriter

Chrissie Hynde
Born 1951, American Pretenders leader

Debbie Harry
Born 1945, American, Blondie frontwoman

Janis Joplin
1943–1970, influential American singer-songwriter and musician

Juliette Lewis
Born 1973, American actor and singer

Karen O
Born 1978, Korean-born singer with the Yeah Yeah Yeahs

Kathleen Hannah
Born 1969, American leader of punk rock movement Riot Grrrl

Patti Smith
Born 1946, American performer and poet

Polly Jean (PJ) Harvey
Born 1969, English singer-songwriter

Siouxsie Sioux
Born 1957, English leader of the Banshees

Singers (Rock)

Axl Rose
Born 1962, American, Guns N' Roses frontman

Bruce Springsteen
Born 1949, American singer-songwriter and instrumentalist, aka 'The Boss'

Chino Moreno
Born 1973, American, Deftones frontman

David Lee Roth
Born 1955, American Van Halen frontman

Elvis Presley
1935–1977, iconic American singer, aka 'The King'

Freddie Mercury
1946–1991, British frontman of Queen

Gene Simmons
Born 1949, American, Kiss frontman

James Hetfield
Born 1963, American, heads up Metallica

Mick Jagger
Born 1943, hip-shaking English Rolling Stone

Sebastian Bach
Born 1968, Canadian, Skid Row frontman

Spies

Belle Boyd
1844–1900, Confederate spy in the American Civil War, aka 'La Belle Rebelle'

Eileen Nearne
1921–2010, English spy in France during World War Two

Elizabeth Van Lew
1818–1900, operated American Civil War spy ring

Krystyna Skarbek
1908–1952, Polish secret agent for the British in World War Two

Lona Cohen
1913–1992, American spy for the Soviet Union

Mata Hari
1876–1917, infamous Dutch World War One spy

Melita Norwood
1912–2005, English spy for the Soviet Union

Nancy Wake
1912–2011, New Zealand-born British wartime spy

Noor Inayat Khan
1914–1944, Russian-born Allied heroine of World War Two

Violette Szabo
1921–1945, French–British secret agent of World War Two

Spies

Aldrich Ames
Born 1941, American CIA agent convicted of spying for the Soviet Union

Anthony Blunt
1907–1983, English art historian and Soviet spy

Donald Maclean
1913–1983, British diplomat and spy for the Soviet Union

Giacomo Casanova
1725–1798, Venetian libertine who spied for the state inquisitors

John André
1750–1780, British Army spy during American War of Independence

Kim Philby
1912–1988, British Intelligence double agent and defector to the Soviet Union

Klaus Fuchs
1911–1988, German–British atomic spy for the Soviet Union

Morton Sobell
Born 1917, American industrial spy for the Soviet Union

Nathan Hale
1755–1776, American Revolutionary War spy hanged by the British

Richard Sorge
1895–1944, German spy for the Soviet Union

Talk Show Hosts

Cilla Black
Born 1943, English singer and entertainer

Joan Rivers
Born 1933, American TV personality and comedian

Oprah Winfrey
Born 1954, American queen of the talk show

Ricki Lake
Born 1968, American actor, producer and TV host

Rosie O'Donnell
Born 1962, American actor, comedian and presenter

Sally Jessy Raphael
Born 1935, American radio and TV presenter

Sharon Osbourne
Born 1952, English music manager, promoter and TV host

Trisha Goddard
Born 1957, English, morning TV host

Tyra Banks
Born 1973, American model and media personality

Vanessa Feltz
Born 1962, English TV personality and journalist

Talk Show Hosts

Conan O'Brien
Born 1963, American comedian and late-night TV host

David Letterman
Born 1947, long-time American talk show host

Graham Norton
Born 1963, Irish comedian and presenter

Jay Leno
Born 1950, American TV host and comedian

Jerry Springer
Born 1944, British-born American host of explosive talk show

Jonathan Ross
Born 1960, English TV personality

Merv Griffin
1925–2007, American TV host and media mogul

Michael Parkinson
Born 1935, legendary English TV host

Montel Williams
Born 1956, American radio and TV personality

Terry Wogan
Born 1938, celebrated Irish radio and TV host

Teachers

Anne Sullivan
1866–1936, Irish-American instructor of Helen Keller

Beatriz Galindo
1465–1534, Spanish physician and teacher

Charlotte Scott
1858–1931, British mathematician and educator

Hallie Quinn Brown
1849–1949, African-American educator, writer and activist

Harriet Beecher Stowe
1811–1896, American abolitionist, author and educator

Inez Prosser
1895–1934, influential African-American teacher

Katharine Lee Bates
1859–1929, American songwriter and English literature professor

Maria Montessori
1870–1952, Italian physician and progressive educator

Mary McLeod Bethune
1875–1955, American educator and civil rights leader

Tilly O'Neill-Gordon
Born 1949, Canadian teacher turned politician

Teachers

Aesop
c.620 BC–c.564 BC, Ancient Greek storyteller and educator

Alexander Sutherland
1883–1973, Scottish founder of the progressive Summerhill school

Andrea del Verrocchio
1435–1488, Italian Renaissance artist and teacher

Confucius
551 BC–479 BC, Chinese philosopher, teacher and politician

Frank McCourt
1930–2009, Irish-American teacher and Pulitzer Prize-winning author

Jaime Escalante
1930–2010, inspirational Bolivian mathematics teacher

Plato
c.424 BC–c.348 BC, Greek founder of first Western school of higher education

Roger Bacon
1214–1294, English philosopher and inspirational teacher

Rudolf Steiner
1861–1925, Austrian lecturer and social reformer

Socrates
c.469 BC–c.399 BC, Greek philosopher and educator

Tennis Players

Arantxa Sánchez Vicario
Born 1971, Spanish Grand Slam winner

Billie Jean King
Born 1943, iconic American player and champion of women's tennis

Chris Evert
Born 1954, American long-running world number one

Jennifer Capriati
Born 1976, American youngest-ever top-ten player

Margaret Court
Born 1942, Australian record breaker

Martina Navratilova
Born 1956, Czech–American tennis legend

Monica Seles
Born 1973, Serbian–American former world number one

Serena Williams
Born 1981, American all-time highest money winner

Steffi Graf
Born 1969, German multiple Grand Slam winner

Venus Williams
Born 1980, American former world number one

Tennis Players

Andre Agassi
Born 1970, American former world number one

Andy Murray
Born 1987, Scottish Olympic gold medallist and Grand Slam winner

Björn Borg
Born 1956, record-breaking Swedish icon

Boris Becker
Born 1967, German six-time Grand Slam winner

Fred Perry
1909–1995, last English player to win Wimbledon

Ivan Lendl
Born 1960, Czech multiple Grand Slam winner

Pat Cash
Born 1965, Australian Wimbledon winner

Pete Sampras
Born 1971, American former world number one

Rafael Nadal
Born 1986, Spanish tennis star

Roger Federer
Born 1981, multiple record-breaking Swiss player

Violinists

Adila Fachiri
1886–1962, inspiring Hungarian violinist

Ethel Barns
1874–1948, English violinist, pianist and composer

Grazyna Bacewicz
1909–1969, Polish composer, violinist and pianist

Guila Bustabo
1916–2002, groundbreaking American violinist

Hélène Jourdan-Morhange
1892–1961, influential French violinist

Jelly d'Arányi
1893–1966, Hungarian violinist and dedicatee of Ravel's 'Tzigane'

Leonora Jackson
1879–1969, world-renowned American violinist

Lillian Shattuck
1857–1940, American, formed first all-female string quartet

Vanessa-Mae Nicholson
Born 1978, convention-defying British violinist

Vivien Chartres
1893–1941, British violin prodigy

Violinists

Antonio Vivaldi
1678–1741, Italian Baroque violinist and composer

Arcangelo Corelli
1653–1713, Italian Baroque violinist

Fritz Kreisler
1875–1962, Austrian violinist and composer

Giuseppe Tartini
1692–1770, Italian Baroque composer and violinist

Itzhak Perlman
Born 1945, Israeli–American violinist and conductor

Jascha Heifetz
1901–1987, Lithuanian–American violin legend

Joshua Bell
Born 1967, American Grammy-winning violinist

Mischa Elman
1891–1967, influential Russian–American violinist

Niccolò Paganini
1782–1840, celebrated Italian violinist and composer

Ole Bull
1810–1880, Norwegian violinist and composer

Writers

Carson McCullers
1917–1967, American Southern Gothic novelist

Charlotte Brontë
1816–1855, English novelist and poet, author of *Jane Eyre*

Doris Lessing
Born 1919, Zimbabwean–British Nobel Prize winner

Harper Lee
Born 1926, American novelist and recluse

Iris Murdoch
1919–1999, Irish-born British author and philosopher

Margaret Atwood
Born 1939, Canadian novelist and poet

Mary Shelley
1797–1851, English creator of *Frankenstein*

Virginia Woolf
1882–1941, English modernist writer

Willa Cather
1873–1947, American famous for her frontier-life novels

Zadie Smith
Born 1975, English novelist, winner of the Orange Prize for Fiction

Writers

Charles Dickens
1812–1870, English novelist and social commentator

Cormac McCarthy
Born 1933, American novelist and playwright

Edgar Allen Poe
1809–1849, American Romantic author and poet

Ernest Hemingway
1899–1961, Nobel Prize-winning American author

Franz Kafka
1883–1924, Austro–Hungarian Modernist novelist

George Orwell
1903–1950, English dystopian novelist and journalist

Jules Verne
1828–1905, pioneering French science-fiction writer

Kazuo Ishiguro
Born 1954, Japanese-born British novelist

Tennessee Williams
1911–1983, Pulitzer Prize-winning American writer

Truman Capote
1924–1984, American Southern Gothic novelist

Writers (Children's)

Angela Sommer-Bodenburg
Born 1948, German creator of The Little Vampire

Beatrix Potter
1866–1943, English creator of Peter Rabbit

Enid Blyton
1897–1968, English creator of The Famous Five

Frances Hodgson Burnett
1849–1924, English writer of *The Secret Garden*

Jacqueline Wilson
Born 1945, English creator of Tracy Beaker

Joanne Rowling
Born 1965, English creator of Harry Potter

Judy Blume
Born 1938, American creator of *Fudge*

Laura Ingalls Wilder
1867–1957, American creator of *Little House on the Prairie*

Louisa May Alcott
1832–1888, American writer of *Little Women*

Shirley Hughes
Born 1927, award-winning English author, introduced us to Alfie

Writers (Children's)

Allan Ahlberg
Born 1938, English writer of the *Please Mrs Butler* poems

Clive (C. S.) Lewis
1898–1963, Northern Irish creator of Narnia

Eric Carle
Born 1929, American creator of *The Very Hungry Caterpillar*

Jacob Grimm
1785–1863, German, one half of Brothers Grimm

Jeff Kinney
Born 1971, American writer of *Diary of a Wimpy Kid*

Kenneth Grahame
1859–1932, Scottish writer of *The Wind in the Willows*

Lewis Carroll
1832–1898, English creator of *Alice in Wonderland*

Philip Pullman
Born 1946, English creator of *His Dark Materials*

Roald Dahl
1916–1990, seminal best-selling British children's author

Wilhelm Grimm
1786–1859, German, other half of Brothers Grimm

Zoologists

Biruté Galdikas
Born 1946, German orangutan specialist

Dian Fossey
1932–1985, American famous for study of gorillas

Ethelwynn Trewavas
1900–1993, English ichthyologist

Eugenie Clark
Born 1922, American shark specialist

Georgina Sweet
1875–1946, Australian zoologist, academic and philanthropist

Helen Gaige
1890–1976, American specialist in Neotropical frogs

Libbie Hyman
1888–1969, American zoologist and natural science author

Roger Arliner Young
1899–1964, African-American zoologist and marine biologist

Sylvia Mead
Born 1935, American oceanographer and aquanaut

Terri Irwin
Born 1964, American-born Australian naturalist and TV presenter

Zoologists

Alfred Kinsey
1894–1956, American zoologist and sexologist

Boyd Alexander
1873–1910, English ornithologist and explorer

David Attenborough
Born 1926, British naturalist and national treasure

Élie Metchnikoff
1845–1916, pioneering Russian protozoologist

Jack Hanna
Born 1947, American zookeeper and TV star

Konrad Lorenz
1903–1989, Austrian Nobel Prize-winning zoologist

Louis-Jean-Marie Daubenton
1716–1800, early French naturalist

Niko Tinbergen
1907–1988, Dutch Nobel Prize-winning ethologist and ornithologist

Steve Irwin
1962–2006, Australian 'Crocodile Hunter'

Tokiharu Abe
1911–1996, Japanese ichthyologist

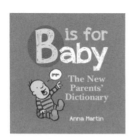

B is for Baby

The New Parent's Dictionary

Anna Martin

£4.99

Hardback

ISBN: 978-1-84953-371-3

M is for Meconium – plutonium, more like. Your baby's first plop is the poo equivalent of rocket fuel and should be disposed of just as carefully.

N is for Nursing bra – easy access for baby, strictly no access for husband.

This tongue-in-cheek dictionary gives you a crash-course in the strange new vocabulary of parenthood, with hilarious observations on everything from the alphabet blocks you will inevitably trip over to the lack of zzz's you will be getting.

New Baby

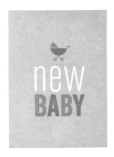

£5.99

Hardback

ISBN: 978-1-84953-372-0

Every baby born into the world is a finer one than the last.

Charles Dickens

What can compare to the miracle of birth? Whether it's their first cry, their tiny little fingers or their gurgles of contentment, nothing compares to the wonder of having a new bundle of joy in the family. This beautiful collection of heartwarming quotes is the perfect gift for anyone welcoming a new baby into the world.

Baby Tips for Mums, Dads and Grandparents

Simon Brett

£4.99

Hardback

ISBNs: 978-1-84953-282-2 (Mums)

978-1-84953-283-9 (Dads)

978-1-84953-284-6 (Grandparents)

Congratulations! After all those months of waiting, your new arrival is finally here, and making its presence felt all over the house – but what happens now?

Whether you're a new parent or you have a PhD in child-rearing, these nifty little books are full of humorous but helpful advice on everything from babysitting to breast pads and will help you through with your nerves and your furniture intact!

Commando Dad:
Basic Training

How to Be an Elite
Dad or Carer

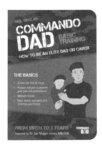

Neil Sinclair

£9.99
Paperback
ISBN: 978-1-84953-261-7

An indispensable training manual for new recruits to fatherhood. Written by ex-Commando and dad of three, Neil Sinclair, this manual will teach you, in no-nonsense terms, how to:

- Plan for your baby trooper's arrival
- Prepare nutritious food for your unit
- Deal with hostilities in the ranks
- Maintain morale and keep the troops entertained

And much, much more.

Let training commence!

If you're interested in finding out more about our gift books, follow us on Twitter: @Summersdale

www.summersdale.com